Study guide to accompany

Psychiatric nursing: contemporary practice

Mary Ann Boyd, PhD, DNS, RN, CS
Professor, Graduate Faculty
Coordinator, Undergraduate Psychiatric Nursing
School of Nursing
Southern Illinois University
Edwardsville, Illinois

Maryann Foley, RN, BSN
Clinical Consultant
Flourtown, Pennsylvania

Lippincott
Philadelphia • New York

Ancillary Editor: *Doris S. Wray*
Acquisition Editor: *Margaret Zuccarini*
Editorial Assistant: *Sara Lauber*
Production Service: *Shepherd, Inc.*
Printer/Binder: *Victor Graphics, Inc.*

ISBN: 0-397-55179-7

Contents

Unit six: Care challenges in psychiatric nursing 131

Appendix A

Answers 170

UNIT ONE
The nature of mental health and mental illness

1 ▪ *The changing perception of mental health*

CHAPTER HIGHLIGHTS

Chapter 1 traces the evolution of mental health from ancient times through present day. It explores the impact of social, political, and religious influences, scientific thought, and social changes on the perception and treatment of the mentally ill.

Chapter 1 key points include the following:

- A combination of socioeconomic and political factors and development of revolutionary ideas often trigger social change.
- Very early in history, mental illness was attributed to being controlled by evil spirits or demons. Patients were viewed as a threat to society, needing to be isolated and removed from society.
- More humane and moral treatments were developed during the 1800s when mental illness began to be viewed as an illness.
- Social reformers, such as Dorothea Dix, Horace Mann, and Clifford Beers have been involved in raising society's awareness and advocating public responsibility for proper treatment of the mentally ill.
- Community mental health centers developed in the twentieth century to offer a wider variety of services, treatment, and follow-up care.
- Scientific thought and psychiatric practice have evolved to include recognition of the importance of the biologic aspect of mental disorders.
- Research in neurobiology has lead to the development of new, more effective psychopharmacologic agents.

STUDENT ACTIVITIES

Matching

Identify the correct description in the righthand column with the correct term in the lefthand column.

_______ 1. Social change
_______ 2. Psychiatric pluralism
_______ 3. Psychosocial theory
_______ 4. Moral treatment
_______ 5. Psychoanalytic movement

a. Belief that environmental and social deprivation results in mental disorders
b. Personality theory based on unconscious motivations for behavior or drives
c. The structural and cultural evolution of society
d. Use of kindness, compassion, and pleasant environment to cure mental illness
e. Integration of human biologic function with the environment

Labeling

Place the letter of the events listed below in the correct location on the time line.

Events:

a. Pennsylvania Hospital established
b. Hill-Burton Act passed
c. First freestanding public asylum established
d. First edition of DSM developed
e. National Health Promotion and Disease Prevention Objectives developed
f. Mental Retardation and Community Mental Health Act signed
g. Chlorpromazine introduced in the United States
h. Abuses at Bicentre in France stopped
i. Moral treatment promoted by Thomas Eddy

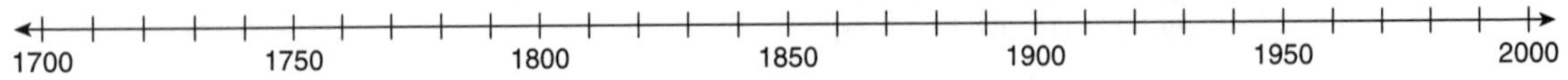

Multiple choice

Circle the option that best answers the question.

1. The belief that mental illness was a result of demonic possession was evidenced by which of the following activities?
   a. Blood letting
   b. Imprisonment
   c. Witch hunts
   d. Corporal punishment
2. Which of the following services were required for funding a community mental health center?
   a. 24-hour emergency care
   b. Follow-up care
   c. Drug abuse services
   d. Elderly services
3. Using Freud's psychoanalytic theory, mental illness occurs as a result of a(n):
   a. Biologic cause
   b. Interference with normal development
   c. Interaction between biologic function and the environment
   d. Environmental and social deprivation
4. The DSM-IV classifies mental illness based on:
   a. Psychoanalytic nomenclature
   b. Psychoses
   c. Subjective symptomatology
   d. Descriptive symptomatology
5. Which of the following statements about contemporary mental health care is true?
   a. The number of community mental health centers currently established exceeded predictions
   b. Costs are being contained through the increased use of inpatient care
   c. States are reducing their mental health expenditures
   d. There is an increasing emphasis on social interactions as a cause of mental illness

6. The antipsychotic medications developed today differ from earlier drugs in that the newer medications:
   a. Have a broader mechanism of action
   b. Cure the mental disorder
   c. Have fewer side effects
   d. Help the patient to be more amenable to treatment

7. Which of thc following incorporates the Healthy People 2000 National Health Promotion and Disease Prevention objectives?
   a. Primary emphasis on treatment, then prevention
   b. Intermittent provision of mental health services
   c. Initial hospitalization followed by community support services
   d. Stress reduction and control

Critical thinking exercises

1. As part of a seminar class, you are assigned to play the role of Dorothea Dix. Develop a speech that illustrates her beliefs and ideas about the mentally ill to present to your classmates.
2. Contact a managed care organization in your area. Investigate how this organization provides for mental health care.
3. Visit a local community mental health center. Analyze the services provided based on those identified and required by the Community Mental Health Construction Act and its amendments.
4. Trace the evolution of treatments for mental illness from the Renaissance through today. Evaluate the pros and cons of each treatment identified.

2 ▪ *Cultural issues related to mental health care*

CHAPTER HIGHLIGHTS

Chapter 2 reviews the impact of culture on mental health care. It explores the various cultural and religious views of mental health, social and economic influences, the "stigma" associated with mental illness, and the changing public attitude toward mental health care, emphasizing the need for cultural competence in psychiatric mental health nursing.

Chapter 2 key points include the following:

- Culture is defined as a way of life manifesting the learned beliefs, values, and accepted behaviors transmitted socially within a specific group.
- Various cultural groups exist in the United States and Canada, each with its own unique values, beliefs, and health care practices.
- While some groups, such as Americans of European descent, have been acculturated into mainstream American culture, some, such as African-American culture, have been segregated.
- Cultural groups and people with mental illness are stigmatized as a result of prejudice, discrimination, and stereotyping. These persons are ostracized by society and view themselves in a negative, demoralizing way.
- As the density of a cultural group decreases, the group's cohesiveness is weakened and members are more exposed to prejudice and less group support.
- Religious beliefs are closely intertwined with beliefs about health and mental illness. In most cultures, mental illnesses are stigmatized as a result of cultural and religious beliefs.
- Poverty and living in rural areas limit access to mental health treatment.
- Traditional health care services need to adapt to meet the mental health care needs of the family, which is rapidly changing in structure, size, and member roles.
- NIMH has initiated campaigns to improve understanding of mental disorders with the goal of reducing the stigma of mental illness. Today families are playing an increasing role as advocates, promoting positive legislative changes.
- Cultural competence consists of cultural awareness, knowledge, skills, and encounters. It is an ongoing process necessary to care for patients within the context of their culture.

STUDENT ACTIVITIES

Word find

Hidden within the following letter grid are key terms from chapter 2, listed below. The terms may be vertical, horizontal, diagonal, or backward. Circle the words as you find them.

Acculturation	Integration
Culture	Prejudice
Cultural competence	Segregation
Group density	Stereotyping
Homophobia	Stigmatization

N	O	T	E	R	O	N	K	S	Y	X	Z	I	M	A	S	I	T	E
I	C	E	D	T	G	I	N	M	E	Y	T	I	D	N	I	E	Y	G
O	R	S	Y	M	P	H	O	C	B	G	I	A	E	G	P	O	U	R
N	I	S	A	O	Z	M	B	U	I	L	R	D	R	N	T	L	C	E
P	A	J	K	H	A	T	R	L	A	S	P	E	N	E	G	I	M	A
E	L	I	T	N	I	U	G	T	R	O	N	S	G	R	D	K	P	O
A	Y	W	E	X	M	N	A	U	U	Y	S	I	T	A	U	T	B	M
Z	P	Z	C	G	A	O	T	R	A	J	N	S	R	C	T	H	O	A
I	D	P	U	R	G	I	G	A	T	B	O	P	N	R	T	I	A	H
M	J	H	D	O	A	T	O	L	R	I	I	E	O	N	M	A	O	L
G	R	O	A	U	P	A	C	C	U	L	T	U	R	A	T	I	O	N
A	C	C	U	P	A	Z	N	O	I	T	A	J	E	R	P	B	A	K
T	U	B	I	D	W	I	W	M	E	A	R	N	B	E	D	O	H	J
S	T	E	R	E	O	T	Y	P	I	N	G	M	R	I	O	H	O	M
E	L	M	A	N	S	P	M	E	L	Z	E	U	S	T	Y	P	I	E
G	R	O	D	S	V	M	K	T	X	M	T	C	U	L	T	O	C	F
R	E	H	B	I	O	G	I	E	Q	L	N	I	A	C	F	M	T	S
A	U	G	C	T	A	I	V	N	U	J	I	U	K	I	O	O	I	T
G	S	D	S	Y	M	T	E	C	I	D	U	J	E	R	P	H	O	L
E	M	A	N	L	I	S	T	E	R	E	O	T	P	P	Y	I	N	G

Fill in the blanks

Read each statement carefully and place your answer in the space(s) provided.

1. ________________ occurs when a minority group assumes the language, beliefs, values, and practices of the predominant culture.
2. Prejudice, discrimination, and stereotyping promote ________________________________.
3. Four dynamics that may account for the group density effect include: ________________; ________________; ________________; and ____________________.
4. In the Mexican-American culture, the __________________ is the most valued institution.
5. In the Korean-American culture, mental illness is viewed as ________________ or caused by ________________.
6. Vietnamese Americans demonstrate respect for ________________ and ________________.
7. In the United States, the size of the family has ________________________________.
8. The stigma attached to homosexuality was intensified with the ____________________________.
9. When subjected to stigmatization over long periods of time, persons begin to ____________ society's ______________ feelings.
10. The National Alliance for the Mentally Ill emphasizes the importance of ____________ factors in the etiology of mental illness.
11. The 1990s have been declared ____.
12. Key to cultural competence is examination of the nurse's own __________________ and ______________.

Multiple choice

Circle the option that best answers the question.

1. When interviewing a patient from an Italian-American family, you find that the patient and his family speak English and have adopted the beliefs and practices of the typical American society. You interpret this family as having been:
   a. Stereotyped
   b. Acculturated
   c. Integrated
   d. Segregated

2. An African-American male employed as a sales representative goes into a local convenience store to pick up some items for dinner. As he walks around the store, the owner sees him and states, "Get out of my store, I'm not going to let you rob me." This is an example of:
   a. Cultural isolation
   b. Dislocation
   c. Prejudice
   d. Discrimination

3. A patient of Mexican-American heritage comes to the community health center. When assessing this patient, it is important to keep in mind which of the following characteristics about his culture?
   a. Emphasis on materialism and competitiveness
   b. Mother as the authority figure
   c. Respect for elderly individuals
   d. Differentiation between physical and emotional illness
4. Which of the following statements is true about the Vietnamese culture?
   a. Tendency to somaticize mental illness
   b. Early treatment of symptomatic behavior
   c. Open disagreement with authority
   d. Increased social support with symptomatic behavior
5. Factors associated with an increase in mental illness include which of the following?
   a. Living within one's own cultural group
   b. Stress of poverty
   c. Urban geographic location
   d. Increase in family size
6. How can the psychiatric nurse provide culturally competent care?
   a. Encourage acculturation
   b. Work with one cultural group
   c. Reinforce segregation
   d. Identify one's own biases
7. When treating a patient who follows the Taoist religion, the nurse understands that this patient believes in which of the following?
   a. Quiet and happy harmony with nature
   b. Worship of God out of love, not fear
   c. Purity and balance in physical and mental life
   d. Human suffering and misery due to desire

Critical thinking exercises

1. As part of a class assignment, you and another student are instructed to role-play the following situation: A Korean-American patient being interviewed by an African-American nurse. Develop a scenario that incorporates culturally competent care.
2. Visit a local community mental health center and interview the administration. Determine the predominant cultural groups serviced by this center and how their needs are addressed.
3. Interview a lesbian family. Explore the various prejudices to which they have been exposed.
4. You are assigned to care for a Latin-American patient. Using the components of culturally competent care depicted below, identify specific actions that may be used to achieve each component. (See Fig. 2–1 in text.)

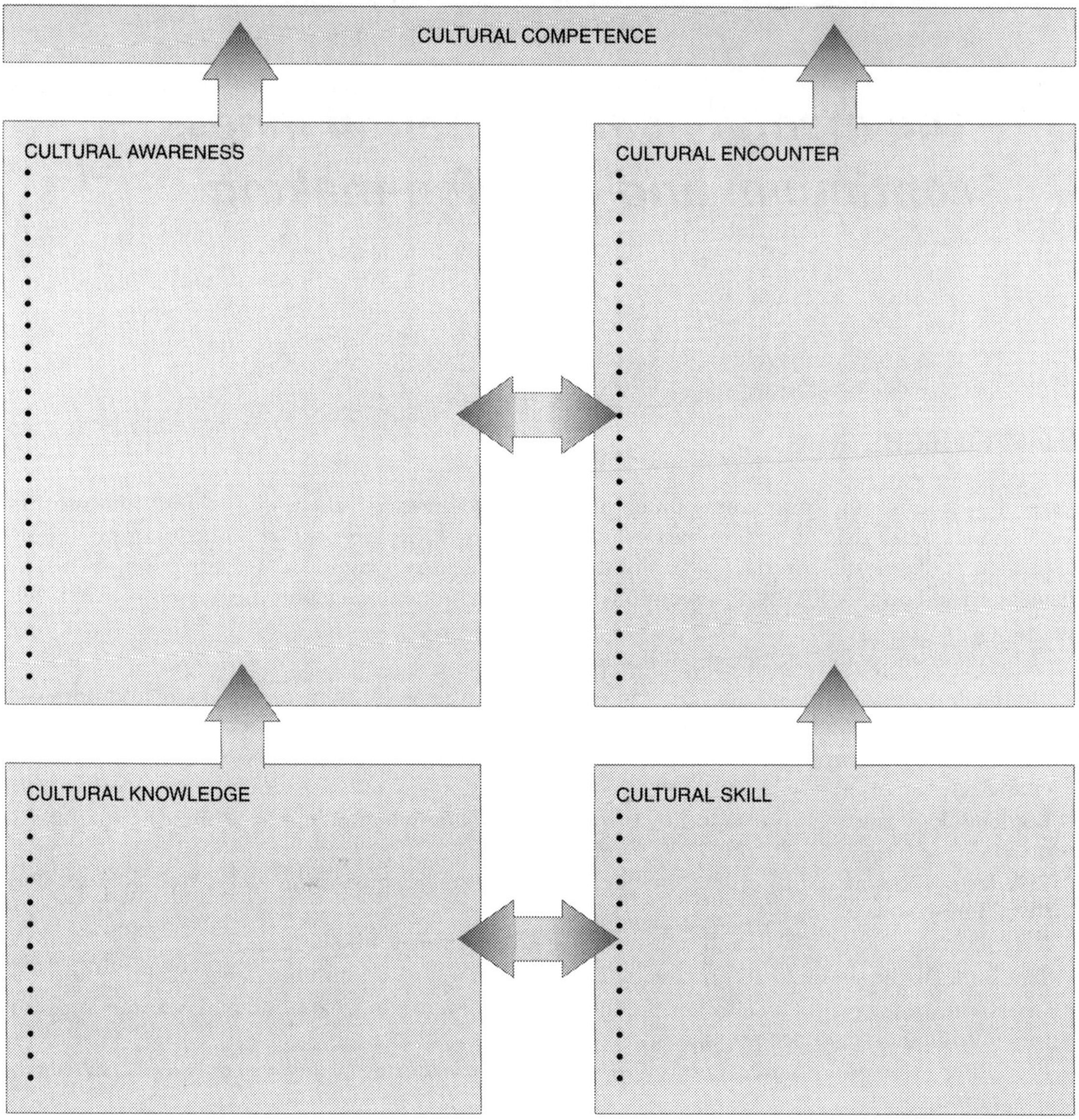
CULTURAL COMPETENCE
CULTURAL AWARENESS
CULTURAL ENCOUNTER
CULTURAL KNOWLEDGE
CULTURAL SKILL

3 ▪ *The mental health—mental illness continuum and decision-making*

CHAPTER HIGHLIGHTS

Chapter 3 examines the continuum of mental health and illness and the use of critical thinking and decision-making in dealing with behaviors and emotions. It explores the complexity of mental illness, such as diagnostic criteria, epidemiology and risk factors, diagnoses and labeling, psychiatric diagnosis based on the DSM IV, interventions, clinical decision-making, and the nurse's role in interdisciplinary care.

Chapter 3 key points include the following:

- Mental disorders imply a separation of mind and body that is antithetical to nursing and does not adequately account for integration of biologic, psychologic, and social aspects.
- Mental illness can be manifest functionality, emotional distress, return of symptoms, and cultural changes.
- Epidemiology assists in understanding the causes, development, and clinical course of mental disorders.
- Risk factors for mental disorders include biologic, genetic, environmental, psychological, and social influences.
- Diagnoses used in mental health may have negative connotations.
- The DSM IV, the standard accepted language in mental health, outlines categorical diagnoses.
- Interventions for mental health may be focused on prevention, treatment, and maintenance for the individual or an entire population.
- Preventive interventions used before the onset of a disorder are categorized as universal, selective, or indicated.
- Formalized critical-thinking tools include the nursing care plan, critical pathway, and algorithm.
- Psychiatric mental health nurses are part of an interdisciplinary team, many times acting as the coordinator in the delivery of care.
- Critical pathways are used throughout the care continuum to ensure quality, cost-effective care.

STUDENT ACTIVITIES

Short answer

Write your answer to the question in the space provided.

1. What factor helps to determine whether a person's reaction is a normal or abnormal psychosocial response?

2. List four areas used to measure mental illness.

3. What term is used to describe long-term mental disorders with periods of exacerbation and remission requiring treatment?

4. Name the three general categories of investigative epidemiologic studies.

5. What is the major obstacle to psychiatric epidemiologic studies?

6. Name two examples of categorical diagnostic systems.

7. What are five characteristics of an ideal critical thinker?

8. What is the primary purpose of the DSM-IV?

9. What are the three goals of Caplan's model of prevention programs?

10. What category of prevention is used to decrease the disability associated with the disorder?

Word unscramble

Below is a list of scrambled words. Unscramble each word and place it in the appropriate space next to its definition.

EYGODIPEMILO	EUCDTEVID HCPPROAA
MIDNEIOSNLA DAGIONESS	EVPEARNECL
SAEX	TSMAGLORHI
SIKR RSFATCO	

1. ______________ Systematic decision trees depicting the flow of decisions and outcomes.
2. ______________ The study of disease distribution patterns in time and space.
3. ______________ Characteristics that increase the likelihood of developing a disorder.
4. ______________ Descriptions of an individual's response to behaviors according to a continuum of degrees ranging from normal to abnormal.
5. ______________ Domains of information.
6. ______________ The total number of persons with a disorder within a given population or a specified time.
7. ______________ Conclusion following stated premises with inferences by reasoning from the general to specific.

Multiple choice

Circle the option that best answers the question.

1. Educating a patient about the need for compliance with his psychopharmacologic therapy regimen is an example of which of the following?
   a. Treatment intervention
   b. Maintenance intervention
   c. Universal preventive intervention
   d. Indicated preventive intervention

2. Which of the following statements by a patient who has experienced a recent stressor of being in a multi-vehicle car accident might indicate an abnormal response?
   a. "I haven't been able to sleep or eat since the accident."
   b. "I've been driving to work every morning."

c. "I'm still playing tennis once a week."
d. "I'm working to get a stoplight installed at that corner."

3. When reviewing a research study about depression, you find that it states that $3/10$ of the general population have experienced depressive symptoms. You identify this statistic as the:
   a. Prevalence
   b. Point prevalence
   c. Rate
   d. Incidence
4. In the DSM IV, where would you expect to find the diagnosis of major depression?
   a. Axis I
   b. Axis II
   c. Axis III
   d. Axis IV
5. After reviewing a patient's chart for information and ascertaining appropriate medical and nursing diagnoses, you devise a possible approach to care. You later confirm this information with your assessment, choosing the most reasonable approach. This is an example of which of the following?
   a. Decision tree
   b. Algorithm
   c. Inductive reasoning
   d. Deductive reasoning
6. When assessing a patient for possible risk factors for psychiatric mental health disorders, you know that which of the following cannot be modified?
   a. Environmental
   b. Genetic
   c. Cultural
   d. Biologic
7. Which of the following statements is true about categorical diagnoses?
   a. Individual responses are described on a continuum
   b. Emotions, such as anger are included
   c. Behaviors are viewed by their degree or severity
   d. Symptoms meet a set of criteria
8. Which step of the decision-making process is the most challenging?
   a. Identifying the clinical decision and the boundaries
   b. Structuring the decision over time
   c. Considering the uncertainties and possible outcomes
   d. Choosing the most appropriate course of action

Critical thinking exercises

1. Compare and contrast the ICD 10, DSM IV, and NANDA nursing diagnoses classification systems. Evaluate the similarities, differences, advantages, and disadvantages of each.

2. You are assigned to care for a newly admitted patient with a panic disorder. Describe how you would use inductive and deductive reasoning to approach the care for this patient.

3. Interview the various members of an interdisciplinary mental health care team in your assigned agency. Examine the roles and functions for each member of the team and evaluate the effectiveness of the care.

4. A 30-year-old female patient, newly admitted to an acute psychiatric unit, is arguing with her roommate about a missing comb and brush. The patient is accusing her of taking it. The patient's anger begins to escalate and she starts to swing her arms wildly toward the roommate. You hear the upset and begin to approach the patient. Using the decision analysis approach shown below, identify the action you need to take to de-escalate the situation.

IDENTIFY THE CLINICAL PROBLEM AND ITS BOUNDARIES

-
-
-
-

↕

STRUCTURE THE DECISION OVER TIME

-
-
-
-

↕

CHARACTERIZE THE INFORMATION NEEDED

-
-
-
-
-
-
-
-

↕

CHOOSE A COURSE OF ACTION

-
-
-
-
-
-
-

4 ▪ *Consumer issues and treatment ethics*

CHAPTER HIGHLIGHTS

Chapter 4 addresses the key legal and ethical issues underlying psychiatric mental health nursing across the care continuum. It explores the issues surrounding consent and confidentiality, the law and psychiatry, protective laws and systems, and ethical frameworks for ethical decision-making.

Chapter 4 key points include the following:

- The right of self-determination allows all patients to refuse treatment, obtain other opinions, and choose other forms of treatment.
- Informed consent must be obtained from a competent individual before any treatment is started to ensure that the information is received and understood.
- Incompetency is court determined when the patient cannot understand the information.
- The right to least restrictive environment protects patients from unnecessary confinement and medication.
- Specialized legal terms and considerations apply to individuals with mental disorders who commit crimes.
- Those determined to be not guilty by reason of insanity demonstrate no understanding of their actions and had no control over them; those guilty but mentally ill applies to those individuals who demonstrate knowledge of the wrongfulness of their actions and had the ability to act otherwise.
- Laws and systems are established to protect the rights of those with mental disorders.
- Specialized departments and agencies within the state mental health system (internal rights protection system) monitor treatment of patients according to the Universal Patient Bill of Rights and state regulations and laws.
- Organizations working outside the state and federal system (external advocacy system) protect the rights of those with mental disorders or handicaps.
- Ethical dilemmas can result from conflicts between the patient's wishes and the opinions of the mental health professional, judgments regarding breach of confidentiality, and overstepping the nurse-patient professional boundaries.
- Knowledge of patients' basic rights and ethical principles guide ethical decision-making.
- Quality of life is commonly used to resolve ethical decisions.

STUDENT ACTIVITIES

Matching

Identify the correct description in the righthand column with the correct term in the lefthand column.

_______ 1. Confidentiality
_______ 2. Competence
_______ 3. Autonomy
_______ 4. Informed consent
_______ 5. Beneficence
_______ 6. Voluntary admission
_______ 7. Involuntary commitment
_______ 8. Intrinsic motivation
_______ 9. Accreditation
_______ 10. Privacy

a. Patient's cognitive ability to process information at a specific time
b. Hospital confinement without the patient's consent
c. Part of a person's life not governed by society's laws and governmental intrusion
d. Ethical duty of nondisclosure
e. Process of judging according to established standards, assuring acceptable quality of care
f. Fundamental right of self-determination
g. Right to determine what shall be done to one's own body
h. Hospitalization with freedom to leave at any time, even if against medical advice
i. Use of science and caring to develop an environment for achievement of maximal care potential
j. Making choices based on personal goals

True/false

Determine whether each sentence below is true or false. If true, write true in the space below. If false, rewrite the sentence to be true.

_______ 1. The patient's right to refuse treatment is based on competency.
_______ 2. A patient giving informed consent is able to communicate choices.
_______ 3. Most states provide for emergency short-term hospitalization of 7 to 10 days.
_______ 4. Guilty but mentally ill individuals are committed to the mental health system.
_______ 5. The American Public Health Association is an example of an internal rights protection system.
_______ 6. The patient has the right to review the records pertaining to his care.
_______ 7. A statistical ethical model bases treatment decisions on the individual's unique situation.
_______ 8. Quality of life issues are viewed in terms of the best interest standard and the relational potential standard.
_______ 9. Self-determinism refers to being empowered, with free will to make moral judgments.
_______ 10. Communication between the patient and mental health care provider is protected by law.

Self-exploration

1. As part of a class simulation, you are interviewing a patient who confides to you that he has been accused of child abuse. He asks you not to tell anyone.
   a. How would you respond?
   b. Identify your feelings toward this patient and his request.
   c. Describe your ethical and legal responsibilities associated with learning this information.

2. Imagine if you were a patient with a terminal illness and were unable to take any foods orally. The physician has ordered you to receive tube feedings.
   a. How would you feel about this?

   b. Would you decide to agree with this intervention and why?

Multiple choice

Circle the option that best answers the question.

1. A patient who decides to seek a second opinion is practicing:
   a. Competency
   b. Informed consent
   c. Self-determinism
   d. Beneficence
2. Placing a patient in restraints before using other methods violates the patient's right to:
   a. Confidential and respectful care
   b. Treatment in a least restrictive environment
   c. Refuse treatment
   d. Provide informed consent
3. A patient who is able to understand what is being explained and can state it in his own words is said to be:
   a. Competent
   b. Autonomous
   c. Incompetent
   d. Logical
4. When is a nurse legally obligated to breach confidentiality?
   a. Anytime the patient is threatening
   b. When the patient violates the nurse's limits
   c. When the patient becomes aggressive
   d. When there is suspicion of harm
5. Accommodation by an employer to meet the needs of a newly hired individual with a mental disorder is established by the:
   a. Health Care Financing Administration
   b. Principles for the Protection of Persons with Mental Illness
   c. Protection and Advocacy for Mentally Ill Individuals Act
   d. Americans with Disability Act
6. A nurse disagrees with the treatment program instituted for a patient diagnosed with aggression. Which of the following is the most appropriate action?
   a. Tell the patient about the disagreement with the treatment program
   b. Evaluate the situation, including the patient's rights and legal aspects
   c. Refuse to participate in the treatment program as planned
   d. Institute an alternative treatment program that meets the nurse's views

Critical thinking exercises

1. Interview a fellow classmate. Evaluate how this individual is self-determined. Support your evaluation with examples of intrinsic and extrinsic motivations for behavior.

2. Obtain a copy of an advanced directive form and complete it. Analyze your feelings about the areas that you identified regarding treatment and nontreatment.

3. A patient with depression is being cared for at home. His family reports that he has been refusing his medications. You note that the patient is becoming increasingly withdrawn, refusing to wash himself, get out of bed, or eat. Can this patient be involuntarily committed? Explain why or why not, providing a rationale for your answer.

UNIT TWO
Principles of psychiatric nursing

5 ▪ The shaping of contemporary psychiatric nursing practice

CHAPTER HIGHLIGHTS

Chapter 5 reviews events that have formed the basis for the unique specialty of psychiatric mental health nursing practice and presents the biopsychosocial model as the organizing framework. It explores the history and development of psychiatric mental health nursing from early views to modern thinking with its integration into mainstream nursing, the impact of legal statutes, professional standards, professional organizations and psychopharmacology, neuroscience, required educational preparation, and development of nursing diagnosis taxonomies.

Chapter 5 key points include the following:

- Even with the recognition of the need for psychiatric mental health nursing near the end of the nineteenth century, much resistance existed toward training women to care for the insane. Training for psychiatric nurses occurred primarily in psychiatric institutions.
- The first nurse organized program of study began in 1913 at Johns Hopkins Phipps Clinic. Gradually all nursing education was phased into generalist nursing education, eventually being incorporated into all diploma and baccalaureate programs.
- Hildegarde Peplau initiated the first graduate program in psychiatric mental health nursing in 1954, preparing nurses for advanced practice.
- Mary Nutting played a key role in establishing nursing practice through a systematic approach based on scientific study and conceptualizing diagnoses, care, and treatment.
- The Standards of Psychiatric Mental Health Clinical Nursing Practice established areas of concerns, standards of care according to the nursing process, and standards of nursing performance, differentiating the functions of the generalist and advanced practice nurse.
- Professional organizations, such as the American Psychiatric Nurses Association, provide leadership in shaping mental health care.
- Psychopharmacologic Guidelines for Psychiatric Mental Health Nurses were formulated by a joint effort of the ANA and NIMH and they describe the basic knowledge necessary for psychopharmacology and skill expectation related to neuroscience, psychopharmacology, and clinical practice.
- Currently, the NANDA taxonomy is endorsed by psychiatric mental health nursing organizations as the standardized classification system. Attempts are being made to integrate the taxonomies of NANDA and DSM IV.
- The biopsychosocial model focuses on three separate, but interdependent, dimensions in the assessment and treatment of mental disorders.

STUDENT ACTIVITIES

Fill in the blanks

Read each statement carefully and place your answer in the space(s) provided.

1. Near the end of the nineteenth century, humane treatment characterizing the ______________ Era was emerging as a model for practice.
2. The first institution in the United States that allowed men to become trained as nurses is ______________.
3. Nightingale viewed the ______________ and ______________ as inseparable.
4. Harriet Bailey wrote the first psychiatric nursing textbook entitled ______________.
5. Hildegarde E. Peplau emphasized the importance of interpersonal relations and the ______________.
6. ______________ are used as guidelines for determining safe acceptable practice.
7. A psychiatric mental health nurse practicing at the basic level holds a ______________ degree in nursing.
8. Promoting the highest professional standards of practice for psychiatric mental health nurses is the primary goal of the ______________.
9. The four stages of psychopharmacologic treatment include: ______________, ______________, ______________, and ______________.
10. NANDA focuses on response ______________; psychiatric mental health nursing system focuses on response ______________.

Labeling

Place the letter of each item below in the appropriate circle on the biopsychosocial diagram.

a. Culture
b. Motivation
c. Fatigue
d. Denial
e. Altered family processes
f. Neurotransmitter activity
g. Awareness of own feelings
h. Altered nutrition
i. Isolation
j. Interpersonal communication
k. Low self-esteem
l. Ethnicity

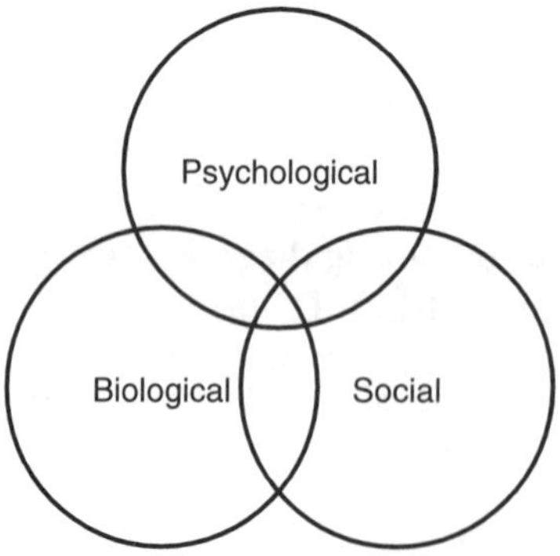

Multiple choice

Circle the option that best answers the question.

1. A psychiatric mental health nurse practicing at the generalist level:
   a. Functions autonomously
   b. Assists patients to regain coping abilities
   c. Performs clinical supervision and consultation
   d. Is a primary mental health care provider

2. Florence Nightingale advocated which of the following?
   a. Care of patients in asylums
   b. Separation of body and soul
   c. Patient dependence on care providers
   d. Patient as a member of the community

3. Which of the following did Peplau identify as the essence of psychiatric mental health nursing?
   a. Nursing care independent of physicians
   b. Nurse's use of self
   c. Nurse-patient relationship
   d. Neurobiologic approach
4. Which of the following is a goal of the APNA?
   a. Collaboration with other groups to influence public policy
   b. Ensurance of access to mental health services for infants and children
   c. Facilitation of excellence in psychiatric mental health nursing
   d. Development of systems to allow sharing of knowledge
5. Which of the following items listed on a patient's chart would the nurse identify as a NANDA nursing diagnosis?
   a. Alprazolam 0.25 mg PO t.i.d.
   b. Major depressive disorder, single episode
   c. Chronic low self-esteem
   d. Problems with primary support
6. Using the biopsychosocial model, the nurse would identify which of the following items listed on a patient's plan of care as a component of the psychological dimension?
   a. Patient lives with parents and younger sister in the city
   b. Patient expresses problems with anger control
   c. Patient sleeps for two hours during the night
   d. Patient verbalizes possible adverse effects of medication
7. To sit for the ANCC generalist certification examination in psychiatric mental health nursing, the nurse must:
   a. Have practiced in direct psychiatric mental health nursing for at least 2000 hours
   b. Have a master's degree in nursing
   c. Currently provide an average of 16 hours per week of direct care
   d. Receive endorsement from a nurse colleague
8. The standards for curriculum development and core competencies used by nursing schools have been established by:
   a. SERPN
   b. ISPCLN
   c. APNA
   d. ANA
9. Before the twentieth century, psychiatric mental health nursing training:
   a. Integrated the concepts of general and mental health nursing
   b. Focused equally on physical and mental care
   c. Was provided in psychiatric institutions
   d. Relied on nurse-authored textbooks

Critical thinking exercises

1. Interview an advanced practice psychiatric mental health nurse. Explore the areas in which this nurse functions and provide specific examples of these functions for each area.

2. Using each of the eight standards of professional performance listed below, describe specific activities that reflect each standard.

Standard	Activities
I. Quality of care	
II. Performance appraisal	
III. Education	
IV. Collegiality	
V. Ethics	
VI. Collaboration	
VII. Research	
VIII. Resource utilization	

3. A patient is prescribed the antidepressant, fluoxetine hydrochloride (Prozac). Using the Psychopharmacology Guidelines for Psychiatric Mental Health Nurses, develop an appropriate plan of care integrating the objectives identified for psychopharmacology.

4. Compare and contrast the goals and functions of APNA, SERPN, and ISCPLN.

6 ▪ *Theoretical basis of psychiatric nursing*

CHAPTER HIGHLIGHTS

Chapter 6 describes the numerous theories providing the basis for psychiatric mental health nursing. It examines biologic, psychological, social, and nursing theories, the research supporting them, and how they are applicable to the psychiatric nursing practice.

Chapter 6 key points include the following:

- The biologic framework forms a new basis for nursing consideration involving such models as general adaptation syndrome, diathesis-stress model, and imbalances in brain chemistry.
- The traditional psychodynamic framework played a role in early nursing interpersonal intervention, such as therapeutic relationships and use of concepts such as transference, countertransference, empathy, and object relations.
- Behavioral theories are often used to help a patient change behavior and thinking.
- Sociocultural theories play a role in understanding and interacting with patients as members of families and cultures.
- Nursing theories, useful in a variety of psychiatric mental health settings, form the conceptual basis for nursing practice.

STUDENT ACTIVITIES

Matching

Identify the theory listed in the righthand column with the correct theorist in the lefthand column.

______ 1. Harry Sullivan	a. Individual psychology
______ 2. Fredrick Perls	b. Analytical psychology
______ 3. Ivan Pavlov	c. General theory of nursing
______ 4. Hans Selye	d. Psychosocial development model
______ 5. Carl Jung	e. Multi-generational family theory
______ 6. Madeleine Lenninger	f. Theory of goal attainment
______ 7. Sigmund Freud	g. Cultural care diversity and universality
______ 8. Imogene King	h. Gestalt therapy
______ 9. Erik Erikson	i. Stimulus response theory
______ 10. Murray Bowen	j. Hierarchy of human needs
______ 11. Jean Watson	k. Theory of unitary human beings
______ 12. Alfred Adler	l. Interpersonal relations theory
______ 13. Abraham Maslow	m. General adaptation syndrome
______ 14. Dorothea Orem	n. Psychoanalytic theory
______ 15. Martha Rogers	o. Theory of the science of caring

Word find

Hidden with the following letter grid are key terms from chapter 6, listed below. The terms may be vertical, horizontal, diagonal, or backward. Circle the words as you find them.

Altruism
Anxiety
Accommodation
Denial
Ego
Empathy
Epigenesis
Family dynamics
Life space
Modeling
Rapport
Role
Self-care
Shaping
Social distance
Transaction
Trust

L	I	F	E	S	P	A	C	E	E	F	I	F	T	E
T	Y	G	R	I	D	N	S	L	N	I	F	R	C	S
P	L	S	Y	S	O	X	O	E	M	R	U	S	M	N
M	I	C	H	E	M	R	C	R	I	S	U	S	A	E
N	C	P	T	N	G	T	I	M	T	R	S	E	E	F
A	M	A	A	E	I	Y	A	O	E	G	G	N	R	D
C	A	K	P	G	N	I	L	E	D	O	M	S	A	M
C	F	A	M	I	L	Y	D	Y	N	A	M	I	C	S
O	N	X	E	P	T	O	I	E	N	Y	D	P	F	I
M	O	D	L	E	U	T	S	T	N	E	C	E	L	U
M	L	O	I	B	J	R	T	R	C	I	E	R	E	R
O	A	X	W	V	O	S	A	O	J	L	A	G	S	T
D	N	E	H	I	R	P	N	P	M	D	N	L	O	L
A	E	P	E	S	P	E	C	N	G	I	R	I	T	A
T	R	E	T	O	D	L	E	M	P	U	W	K	C	N
I	O	C	R	A	M	O	L	A	F	A	B	E	S	D
O	J	T	P	R	A	T	H	I	E	O	N	L	I	C
N	O	I	T	C	A	S	N	A	R	T	Z	A	T	A

Short answer

Write your answers in the space provided.

1. Describe the two concepts involved with the diathesis-stress model.

2. Name the three parts of the personality identified by Freud.

3. Identify the underlying concept of the school of individual psychology.

4. Describe the two types of neuroses identified by Horney.

5. Explain how Sullivan's theoretical approach differs from Freud's approach.

6. List the two concepts developed by Carl Rogers.

7. Describe the two views of countertransference.

8. Identify the defense mechanism illustrated by each of the following examples:
   a. "I really don't love him. We were just on two different career tracts and we didn't see eye to eye on anything that was important."

   b. An angry employee slams the door after a confrontation with his employer.

   c. "I'm not the one who is jealous of your good looks. You're jealous of me."

   d. "I'm not upset that he lost all that money on gambling on football. Betting on football is fine."

   e. A woman who was abused as a young child becomes extremely anxious when returning to the house where the abuse occurred.

   f. "I haven't heard back about my interview results yet. Let's go shopping."

   g. An elderly man, previously independent, becomes rude and shouts obscenities to his full-time caretakers.

9. Name the two major concepts associated with John Watson's theory.

10. Explain Piaget's view of intelligence.

11. State the primary focus of Bowen's theory.

12. List the three phases of the professional relationship as identified by Peplau.

13. Name the concept used by Travelbee to describe the way nurses perceive and relate to other human beings.

14. Identify the goal of nursing care as described by Sister Callista Roy.

15. Explain the rationale for using Orem's theory in psychiatric mental health nursing.

Multiple choice

Circle the option that best answers the question.

1. A patient's behavior reveals difficulty controlling sexual desire. Using Freud's psychoanalytic theory, the basis for this problem is associated with which of the following?
   a. Superego
   b. Ego
   c. Id
   d. Libido
2. According to Adler's beliefs, the second child of a family typically demonstrates which of the following behaviors?
   a. Cooperation with others
   b. Concerns about authority issues
   c. Lack of competitiveness
   d. Protection of others
3. Providing for patient privacy during a physical exam helps to meet which of the following needs?
   a. Physiologic
   b. Safety and security
   c. Love and belonging
   d. Esteem
4. A patient diagnosed with terminal breast cancer screams at the physician saying, "You should have found this earlier." The patient is using which of the following?
   a. Denial
   b. Displacement
   c. Idealization
   d. Rationalization
5. A patient receives a pink slip each time he participates in the unit's activities. Later, he uses these to purchase a snack. This technique is based on the work of:
   a. Lewin
   b. Watson
   c. Skinner
   d. Bandura
6. A person who doesn't smoke marijuana is at a party with a group of friends. He sees his friends smoking marijuana and joins in. This person is exhibiting:
   a. Operant behavior
   b. Shaping
   c. Respondent behavior
   d. Disinhibition
7. The nurse asks a child to arrange a group of blocks from smallest to largest to assess the child's intellectual development. The child does so correctly. Using Piaget's theory, the nurse determines that this child is in which stage of development?
   a. Sensorimotor
   b. Preoperational
   c. Concrete operations
   d. Formal operations
8. Interacting with a patient to identify available resources within the patient's community and culture to meet biologic needs reflects which of the following nursing theorist's beliefs?
   a. Hildegarde Peplau
   b. Imogene King
   c. Joyce Travelbee
   d. Jean Watson
9. When assessing a patient, the nurse views the patient as an open system and identifies variables such as geographic location and expectations, as impacting on the patient's health status. The nurse is using which of the following nursing theories/ models as the foundation?
   a. Science of caring
   b. Theory of unitary human beings
   c. Theory of goal attainment
   d. Adaptation model
10. Which of the following activities would the nurse do when applying Orem's general theory of nursing?
    a. Focus on the patient's encounter with stress
    b. Instruct the patient about his medications
    c. React to the patient's behavior
    d. Find meaning in the patient's suffering

Critical thinking exercises

1. Compare and contrast the major concepts of the psychodynamic and behavioral theories. Evaluate their strengths and weaknesses for use in psychiatric mental health nursing of today.

2. A 23-year-old male is enrolled as a full-time nursing student. He just began his clinical rotations this semester. He lives at home with his parents and two younger siblings. Although he has his own room, he often helps the younger siblings with their schoolwork, doing his studying after everyone is asleep. He also works 20 hours/week as a cashier. Recently he has been falling asleep in class and skipping breakfast and lunch to study and prepare for clinical assignments. Most nights he sleeps five hours or less. Using Maslow's theory, identify this person's priority needs and develop strategies to help him meet these needs.

3. Look back on a time when you were under stress. Analyze your reactions using Selye's general adaptation syndrome.

4. As part of a class assignment, you are required to research a nursing theorist of your choice. Explain why you chose this particular theorist and develop arguments for and against accepting this theorist's beliefs.

7 ▪ *The biologic foundations of psychiatric nursing*

CHAPTER HIGHLIGHTS

Chapter 7 describes the information necessary for a basic understanding of neuroscience as it relates to psychiatric mental health nursing and integration of the biopsychosocial model. It explores neuroanatomy and neurophysiology of the CNS including support structures, nerve impulses, receptors and neurotransmitters, new fields of study, and diagnostic methods for studying CNS and behavior.

Chapter 7 key points include the following:

- Several approaches, such as comparative, developmental, cytoarchitecture, chemoarchitecture, and functional, may be used to study the CNS.
- Behavior and cognitive function are believed to result from complex interactions within the CNS and its ability to adapt to change (plasticity).
- The left hemisphere of the brain is associated with verbal language, verbal learning and memory, temporal order and sequencing, and numerical symbols.
- The right hemisphere of the brain is more associated with nonverbal input, nonverbal learning and memory, spatial orientation and recognition, speech intonation and aspects of music, and facial recognition and emotion.
- Each hemisphere is divided into four lobes: frontal, parietal, temporal, and occipital.
- The frontal lobe controls motor speech function, personality and working memory; the parietal lobe controls sensory function; the temporal lobe contains primary olfactory and auditory areas; the occipital lobe controls visual integration of information.
- Limbic system structures are involved in memory and emotional behavior. Dysfunction here has been linked to schizophrenia, depression, and anxiety disorders.
- Neurons communicate through synaptic transmission. Neurotransmitters, which excite or inhibit a response at a receptor site, have been linked to certain mental disorders.
- New fields of biologic study include psychoendocrinology, psychoimmunology, and chronobiology.
- Biologic markers, physical indicators of disturbances in the CNS differentiating one disease from another, are measured by methods such as challenge tests, EEG, polysomnography, EP, CT scanning, MRI, PET, and SPECT.
- Significant evidence indicates a possible genetic predisposition for several psychiatric disorders. Thus risk factor identification is crucial for planning interventions to prevent development of a disorder or prevent certain behavior patterns.

STUDENT ACTIVITIES

Labeling

1. On the illustration below, identify the following functional areas.

Broca's area
Motor cortex
Primary auditory area
Primary visual area
Wernicke's area

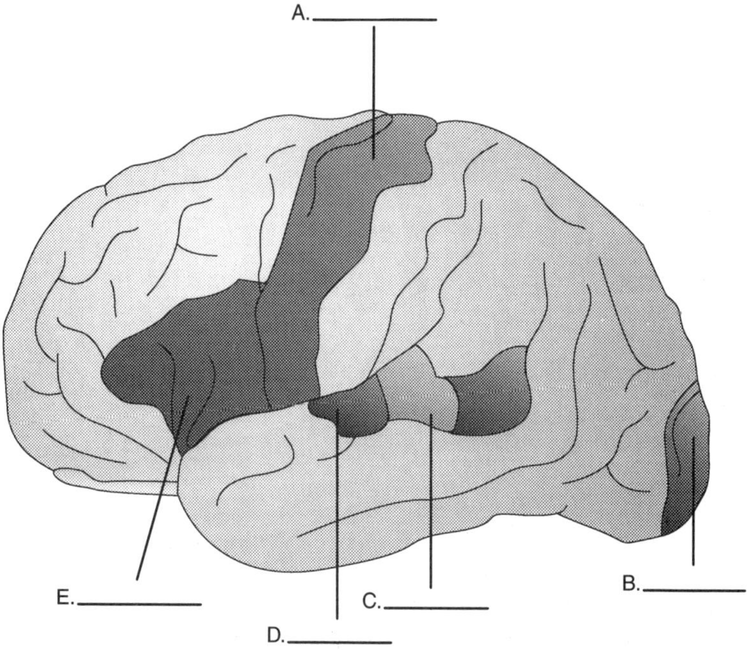

2. On the illustration below, identify the following structures.

Brainstem
Corpus callosum
Cerebellum
Diencephalon
Frontal lobe
Limbic lobe
Occipital lobe
Parietal lobe

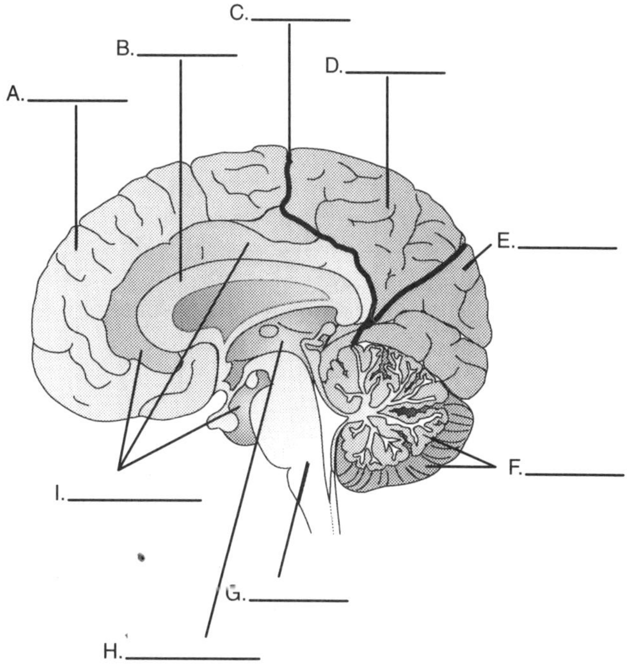

3. On the illustration below, identify the following structures of the limbic system and surrounding area.

Amygdala	Mammillary bodies
Cingulate gyrus	Pituitary
Fornix	Septum
Hippocampus	Thalamus

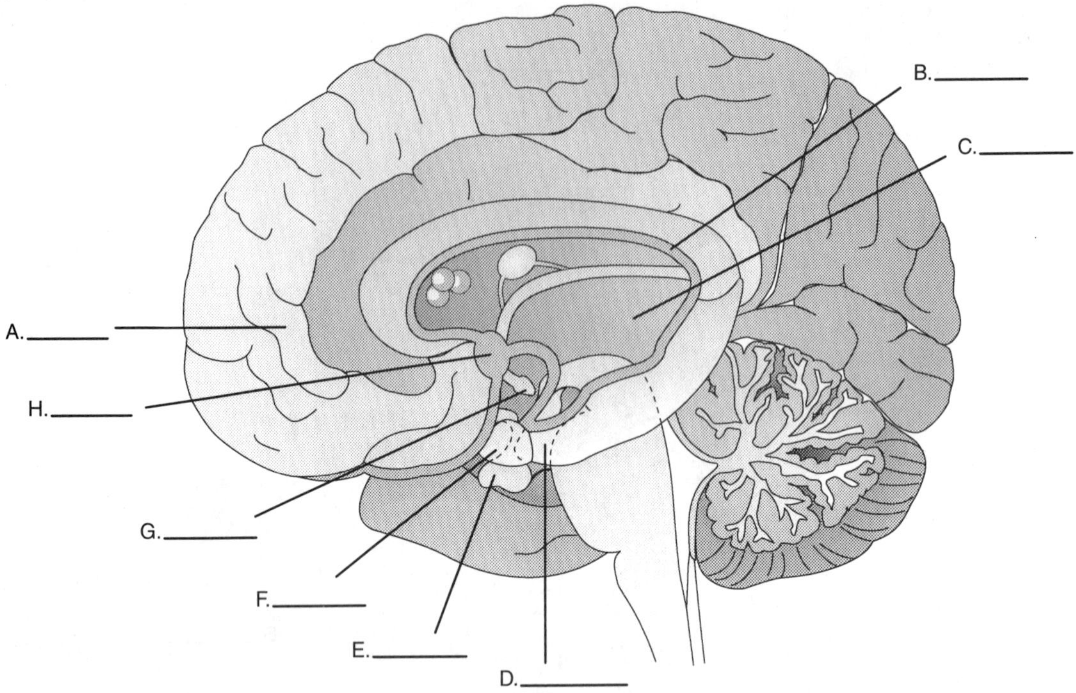

Fill in the blanks

Read each statement carefully and place your answer in the space (s) provided.

1. The ______________ cushions the brain and is produced in the ______________ within each ventricle.
2. The ______________ approach identifies variations in cell type, structure, and density throughout the brain.
3. The brain's ability to change and compensate for functional loss is termed ______________.
4. Shallow grooves of the cortex are called ______________; deeper grooves are called ______________.
5. The ______________ separates the posterior boundary of the frontal lobe from the parietal lobe.
6. Embedded in each temporal lobe is the ______________, which contributes to memory.
7. The brain stem includes the ______________, ______________, and ______________.
8. Located within the hindbrain, the ______________ is primarily responsible for inducing sleep.
9. Most neurons have only one ______________ and numerous ______________.
10. The influx of ______________ ions stimulates the release of neurotransmitters.
11. The main neurotransmitter of the peripheral nervous system is ______________.
12. Biologic rhythms are set by ______________.
13. Monitoring a patient's biologic response to the administration of a chemical known to produce a specific set of symptoms is called a ______________.
14. With EEG, a normal awake adult has mostly ______________ activity with eyes closed, ______________ activity with eyes open, and no ______________ or ______________ activity.

15. For each of the following responses, identify whether it is the result of sympathetic or parasympathetic innervation.
   a. Bronchoconstriction ______
   b. Contraction of bladder sphincter ______
   c. Increased sweat gland secretion ______
   d. Increased GI motility ______
   e. Increased cardiac contractility ______
   f. Vasodilation ______
   g. Pupillary dilation ______

Multiple choice

Circle the option that best answers the question.

1. A patient exhibits twitches and tremors. The nurse understands that the patient may have damage to his:
   a. Temporal lobe
   b. Basal ganglia
   c. Cortex
   d. Broca's area
2. When reviewing a patient's chart, the nurse reads that the patient has suffered damage to Wernicke's area. The nurse anticipates that this patient will probably have difficulty with:
   a. Comprehending speech
   b. Articulating speech
   c. Remembering recent events
   d. Controlling his emotions
3. A patient is diagnosed with seasonal affective disorder requiring exposure to light to relieve the symptoms. The nurse understands that the light is considered which of the following?
   a. Risk factor
   b. Association
   c. Neurotransmitter
   d. Zeitgeber
4. While studying for an examination on neurohormones, the nurse correctly identifies melatonin as being associated with which of the following?
   a. Appetite
   b. Sleep
   c. Smooth muscle contraction
   d. Memory
5. A patient is diagnosed with an injury to the lower portion of the pons. When caring for the patient, the nurse would expect to monitor which of the following?
   a. Pupillary constriction to light
   b. Head movement in response to sound
   c. Respiratory rate and regulation
   d. Deep tendon muscle reflexes
6. While reading, a student sees an illustration of a coronal section of the brain. The student is viewing the structures as they would be seen from the:
   a. Front
   b. Rear
   c. Top
   d. Side
7. A patient is scheduled for SPECT testing. To prepare the patient, the nurse understands that this test evaluates:
   a. Brain wave activity recorded during sleep
   b. Electrical brain activity in response to stimulation
   c. Brain and skull structures using serial X rays
   d. Cerebral blood flow using radioisotopes
8. When planning interventions for the patient with Alzheimer's disease, it is important to remember that the nerves primarily affected involve the:
   a. Amygdala
   b. Hippocampus
   c. Limbic system
   d. Pineal body
9. Substances that increase the cell membrane's susceptibility to the effects of the primary neurotransmitter are termed:
   a. Neuromodulators
   b. Neurohormones
   c. Neuropeptides
   d. Neuroreceptors
10. Which of the following is responsible for accommodation necessary for near vision?
    a. Norepinephrine
    b. Dopamine
    c. Acetylcholine
    d. Serotonin

Critical thinking exercises

1. As part of a class discussion group, you are assigned to present information about the proposed function of the neurotransmitter, serotonin. Develop an outline of your presentation for your fellow students that addresses this topic.

2. Imagine if a friend asks you to participate in an adult education class dealing with the biology of psychiatric disorders. The class is composed of men and women who work as aides and technicians in the local community mental health system. Your role is to review the neuroanatomy and neurophysiology of the CNS. Develop a teaching plan appropriate for this group.

3. Compare and contrast the current structural and functional neuro-imaging techniques, including patient preparation, uses, techniques, advantages, and disadvantages.

8 ▪ *The basics of biologic treatments*

CHAPTER HIGHLIGHTS

Chapter 8 describes the use of psychopharmacologic and somatic therapies in the treatment of psychiatric and mental illness. It reviews the foundational concepts of drug pharmacodynamics, pharmacokinetics, and phases of treatment. The chapter explores the major categories of agents used, including antipsychotics, antimania, antidepressants, antianxiety and sedative-hypnotic agents, and psychostimulants, as well as other forms of biologic treatment, such as electroconvulsive therapy, light and nutritional therapies. It also examines the psychosocial issues often associated with these therapies.

Chapter 8 key points include the following:

- Psychopharmacology, the study of medications used to affect the brain and behavior in the treatment of psychiatric disorders, includes antipsychotics, mood stabilizers (antimania), antidepressants, antianxiety medications, and psychostimulants.
- Pharmacodynamics, the study of drug action on tissues and the human body, has focused on specific actions at receptor sites, ion channel sites, enzyme actions, and carrier proteins.
- Current belief is that the biologic action of each drug depends on how its structure interacts with a specific receptor, functioning as an agonist or antagonist.
- Three qualities determine a drug's ability to interact with a given receptor type: selectivity, affinity, and intrinsic activity.
- Specific drug characteristics affect how well they act and how they affect the patient. Familiarity with these characteristics is crucial for medication administration and patient education to ensure safety and encourage compliance.
- Pharmacokinetics, the study of how the human body processes the drug, involves absorption, distribution, metabolism, and elimination. Bioavailability, the amount of drug that actually reaches circulation through the body, varies widely among individuals based on physiologic differences, such as age, genetic makeup, other disease processes, and chemical interactions.
- Antipsychotic medications, used to treat psychotic disorders, act primarily by blocking dopamine or serotonin postsynaptically. Because of the number of actions on other neurotransmitters, these medications have many side effects.
- Medication-related movement disorders, a serious group of side effects primarily associated with antipsychotic agents, may be acute syndromes, such as dystonia, pseudoparkinsonism, and akathisia, or chronic syndromes, such as tardive dyskinesia.
- Mood stabilizers (antimania medications) are used to control wide variations in mood related to mania and to treat other disorders. Lithium and anticonvulsants are chemically unrelated and act in different ways to stabilize mood.
- Antidepressant medications, varying in structure and action, act by blocking reuptake of one or more of the bioamines, especially serotonin and norepinephrine. Selective serotonin reuptake inhibitors, newer antidepressants, have fewer side effects and are less lethal in overdose than the older tricyclic antidepressants.
- Antianxiety medications, benzodiazepines and non-benzodiazepines, are principally used in psychiatry. Benzodiazepines act by enhancing the effects of GABA while non-benzodiazepine, buspirone, acts on serotonin.
- Psychostimulants, most often used for treatment of symptoms related to attention deficit hyperactivity disorder or narcolepsy, enhance neurotransmitter activity by acting on a number of sites in the nerve.

- ECT involves application of an electrical pulse stimulus to induce seizures in the brain. Neurotransmission is affected resulting in rapid relief of symptoms of depression.
- Phototherapy, application of full spectrum light in the morning hours, appears to reset circadian rhythm delays related to seasonal affective disorder and other forms of depression.
- Compliance, the ability of the individual to self-administer medications as prescribed and to follow other instructions related to medication treatment, can be affected by a number of factors, such as side effects, denial of illness, stigma and family influences, resulting in noncompliance. Nurses play a crucial role in educating patients and helping them to improve compliance.

STUDENT ACTIVITIES

Labeling

1. Each illustration drawn below depicts the location of a major neurotransmitter and its pathway. Place the name of the appropriate neurotransmitter involved in the space provided.

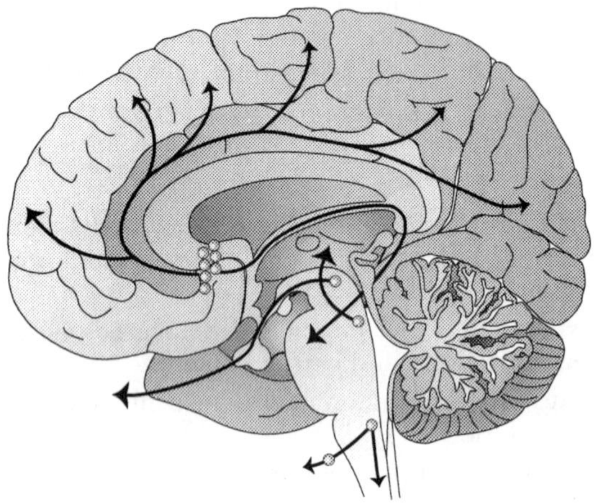

a. ____________________

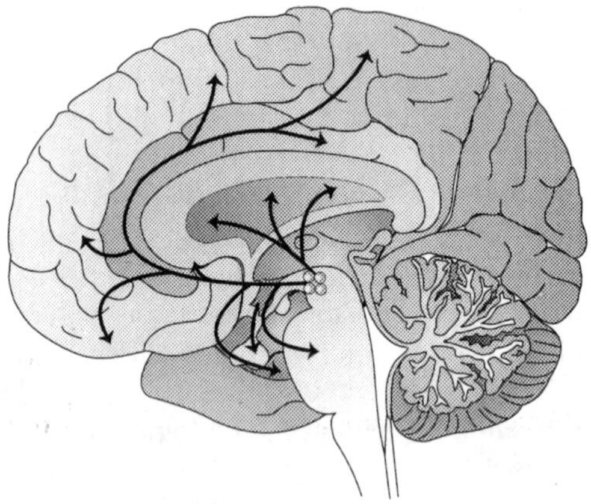

b. ____________________

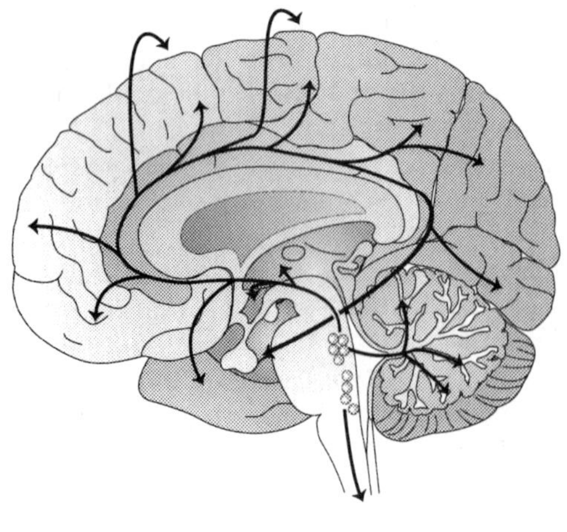

c. ____________________

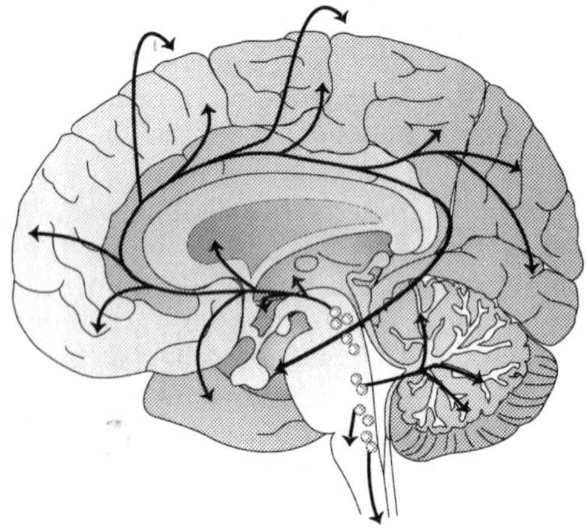

d. ____________________

2. Each of the drugs listed below have a high affinity for receptor blockade or reuptake inhibition of a specific neurotransmitter. Using the illustrations from # 1(above), place the letter(s) of the illustration depicting the neurotransmitter involved next to the correct drug.

a. Buproprion ______________________________

b. Clozapine ______________________________

c. Trazodone ______________________________

d. Desipramine ______________________________

e. Fluoxetine ______________________________

f. Haloperidol ______________________________

g. Amitryptyline ______________________________

h. Thioridazine ______________________________

i. Yohimbine ______________________________

Crossword puzzle

Across

2. Medications affecting the brain and behavior
5. Drug blocking the response at a receptor
7. Gradual dosage reduction
8. Impaired muscle tone
10. Receptor occupancy by a drug for a response
11. Drug amount found at target organ site of action
12. Harmful bloodstream drug concentration
13. Drug's specificity for a receptor

Down

1. Exposure to artificial light source
2. Biologic action of drugs on living tissue
3. Area where specific chemical reacts
4. Drug acting like the neurotransmitter
6. Inability to sit still
9. Degree of attraction between drug and receptor

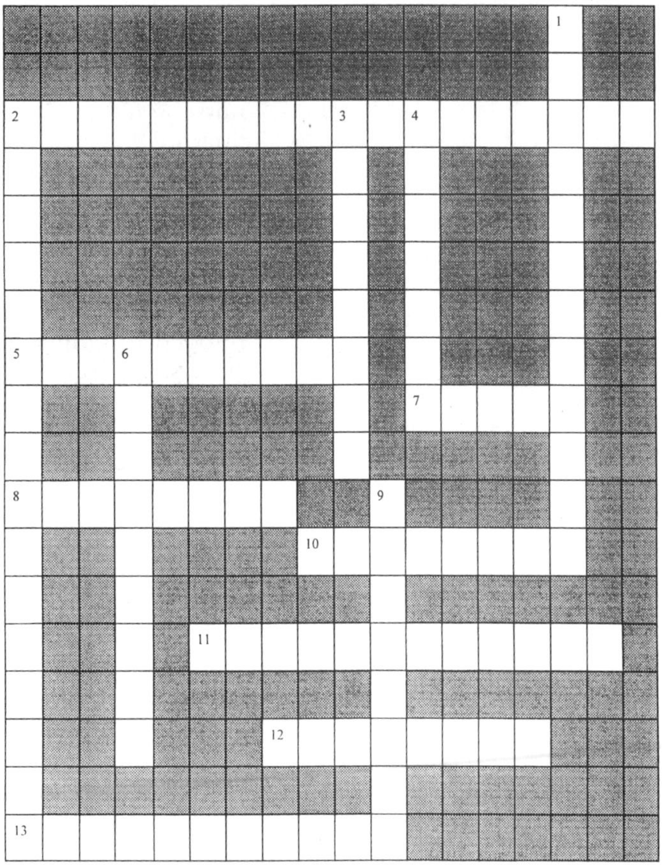

Multiple choice

Circle the option that best answers the question.

1. A patient who has been compliant with his benzodiazepine therapy regimen for treatment of anxiety over the past few months begins to complain of increasing symptoms of anxiety. Assessment reveals no evidence of other possible contributory factors for the increase in symptoms. The nurse strongly suspects that which of the following is occurring?
   a. Toxicity
   b. Tolerance
   c. Selectivity
   d. Desensitization
2. A acutely suicidal patient with major depressive syndrome is prescribed fluoxetine. The nurse understands the rationale for using this drug in this situation is based on which of the following?
   a. High therapeutic index
   b. Minimal risk for side effects
   c. Low incidence of tolerance
   d. High affinity for dopamine receptors
3. The nurse is preparing to administer an oral concentrated form of thioridazine (Mellaril) to a patient. The nurse should choose which of the following liquids to dilute and administer the drug?
   a. Prune juice
   b. Milk
   c. Water
   d. Cranberry juice
4. A patient initially prescribed an antidepressant shows only partial improvement in his symptoms. As a result, the physician orders a mood stabilizer to enhance the effects. The nurse identifies this action as which of the following?
   a. Polypharmacy
   b. Stabilization
   c. Augmentation
   d. Treatment resistance
5. Patient assessment reveals delusions, hallucinations, bizarre ideation, and blunted affect. The nurse anticipates a physician order for which of the following?
   a. Mood stabilizer
   b. Antidepressant
   c. Antipsychotic
   d. Anxiolytic
6. The physician orders chloropromazine for a patient who is also taking hydrochlorothiazide for treatment of hypertension. Based on the nurse's knowledge of possible drug interactions, the nurse should monitor the patient for which of the following?
   a. Hypertensive crisis
   b. Increased sedation
   c. Decreased extrapyramidal symptoms
   d. Severe hypotension
7. Which of the following patients would the nurse identify as being at increased risk for tardive dyskinesia?
   a. 35-year-old male with brain damage
   b. 55-year-old female with depression
   c. 60-year-old male receiving short-term antipsychotic therapy
   d. 40-year-old female on high dose antipsychotic therapy
8. A patient is scheduled to receive haloperidol by depot injection. When administering the drug, the nurse should do which of the following?
   a. Administer it by Z-track technique
   b. Use a 22 gauge or smaller needle
   c. Massage the injection site vigorously
   d. Wait 30 minutes after preparing the syringe and medication
9. When monitoring lithium blood levels, the nurse would expect to have the specimen drawn:
   a. 1 hour before the next dose
   b. 1 hour after the next dose
   c. 12 hours after the next dose
   d. Every other day
10. A patient with bipolar disorder does not respond to lithium therapy, so the physician orders carbamazepine. The patient also is extremely malnourished from loss of appetite, lack of food intake, irritability, and hyperactivity. The nurse would be alert for which of the following?
    a. Stabilized drug plasma levels
    b. Increased incidence of side effects
    c. Increased drug absorption
    d. Relapse in symptoms
11. Which of the following agents has the quickest onset of action after one dose?
    a. Triazolam
    b. Chlordiazepoxide
    c. Chlorazepate
    d. Diazepam

12. When evaluating the teaching plan for a patient receiving a tricyclic antidepressant, which of the following statements by the patient indicates the need for additional teaching?
    a. "I'll make sure to refill my prescription before I run out of pills."
    b. "I'll sit on the edge of the bed for a few minutes before I get up."
    c. "I'll chew some sugarless gum if my mouth gets dry."
    d. "I'll wait 5 to 10 minutes before I drive my car."
13. When studying for an examination about benzodiazepines, the student demonstrates understanding of their mechanism of action by identifying which of the following?
    a. Potentiates the effect of GABA
    b. Interferes with sodium-potassium pump
    c. Blocks reuptake of dopamine
    d. Releases catecholamines
14. When caring for a patient who is prescribed methlyphenidate, the nurse would expect the patient to exhibit possible side effects within what time period after starting therapy?
    a. 24 to 48 hours
    b. 1 to 2 weeks
    c. 2 to 3 weeks
    d. 4 to 5 weeks
15. The nurse would anticipate which of the following treatments for the patient with severe depression?
    a. Phototherapy
    b. Electroconvulsive therapy
    c. Tryptophan supplements
    d. Megavitamin therapy

Critical thinking exercises

1. The drug, trifluoperazine (Stelazine), 10 mg b.i.d., is ordered for a patient who is to be discharged to his family. Develop a teaching plan for the patient and his family incorporating the important information about this drug.

2. In your clinical area, review the charts of several patients for the pharmacologic agents prescribed.
    a. Do you notice any significant patterns about the agents prescribed? If so, please explain.

    b. For each of these agents, propose a rationale for its use for this patient rather than another agent.

3. Common reasons for medication noncompliance are listed in the chart below. Suggest at least 3 nursing interventions for each reason from integration of your knowledge of psychopharmacology that would be helpful in overcoming the noncompliance.

Reason for noncompliance	*Possible nursing interventions*
Uncomfortable side effects	
Side effects interfering with quality of life	
Lack of awareness or denial of illness	
Stigma	
Feeling better	
Confusion about dosage or timing	
Difficulties in access to treatment	
Substance abuse	

4. Imagine if you and a fellow classmate were asked to role-play the following situation. A patient with schizophrenia receiving antipsychotic medications develops acute extrapyramidal symptoms. One of you is to assume the role of the patient. The other is to play the nurse. However, you won't know which role you are to play until the instructor tells you in class the next day.
   a. In preparing for this class, describe the specific areas that need to be addressed for each role.

   b. Create a possible scenario including strategies that demonstrate synthesis of these important areas identified above.

UNIT THREE
Contemporary psychiatric nursing practice

9 ▪ *Communication and the therapeutic relationship*

CHAPTER HIGHLIGHTS

Chapter 9 reviews the nurse-patient relationship using Peplau's model as a tool for intervention. It explores the need for self-awareness in the biological, psychological, and social dimensions, use of therapeutic communication, and important concepts, such as rapport, empathy, boundaries, and zones in the therapeutic nurse-patient relationship.

Chapter 9 key points include the following:

- Self-awareness of one's own cultural values, beliefs, and interpersonal strengths and limitations is crucial for establishing a therapeutic nurse-patient relationship.
- Therapeutic communication, including verbal and nonverbal methods, are used to focus the relationship on therapeutic questions and the patient's problems.
- Communication skills include active listening, positive body language, appropriate verbal responses, and ability to appropriately interpret and analyze the patient's verbal and nonverbal behaviors.
- Behaviors, such as avoiding difficult issues or reacting defensively to unpleasant behaviors and comments, block communication and undermine the therapeutic relationship.
- Certain physical, emotional, and social boundaries and limitations are required in the nurse-patient relationship. Too much self-disclosure, establishing "friendships" with patients, or fostering an unhealthy level of patient dependence should be avoided.
- Empathy and establishing rapport with patients to make them feel understood and accepted are two of the most important guiding principles of the nurse-patient relationship.
- Peplau's model involves three major overlapping phases—orientation (patient and nurse meet and establish parameters of the relationship), working (patient identifies problems and explores them), and resolution (patient learns to manage the problems and relationship ends).
- Specific boundaries and parameters including time limits are established with the first meeting between the patient and the nurse. These parameters are discussed with the patient and agreed on in a verbal contract.

STUDENT ACTIVITIES

Word unscramble

Below is a list of scrambled words. Unscramble each word and place it in the appropriate space next to its definition.

FSLE SEWERANSA	VRAEBL MOUCTMCNAION
SMEETH	RPPORAT
YMATHEP	MSOIMYBLS
ONDBUAISRE	ESLTIROUON
EABRVL TCTOCNRA	RFETONLECI

1. ________________ Gestures, expressions, and body language used during an interaction.
2. ________________ Using words or phrases to represent an object, event, or feeling
3. ________________ Final phase of the nurse-patient relationship.
4. ________________ Limits of a person, object, or relationship.
5. ________________ Interpersonal harmony characterized by understanding and respect.
6. ________________ Redirecting an idea back to the patient.
7. ________________ Understanding own beliefs, thoughts, motivations, biases, and limitations with recognition of how they affect interaction with others.
8. ________________ Discussing responsibilities of nurses and patient along with other parameters on the first visit.
9. ________________ Putting one's self into another's circumstances and feelings.
10. ________________ Repeated expressions of concerns or feelings in several different ways.

Self-exploration

1. Using the questions listed in text box 9-1, evaluate your own cultural heritage. After answering these questions, evaluate your responses in light of their effect on forming an effective nurse-patient relationship. For those areas that are detrimental, propose possible strategies to improve them.

2. Analyze your four body space zones. Explore your reactions when someone violates each of these zones.

3. Using table 9-5, rate your boundary index. For those statements where you responded "sometimes" or "often," explore possible methods to decrease your vulnerability.

Multiple choice

Circle the option that best answers the question.

1. When developing a verbal contract with a patient, the nurse includes which of the following?
   a. Problem identification
   b. Community referrals
   c. Patient responsibilities
   d. Strategy development

2. During termination, a patient displays anger at the nurse. Which of the following responses by the nurse is most therapeutic?
   a. "You shouldn't feel angry. Look how hard you have worked."
   b. "It's okay to feel angry. Anger is a normal emotion."
   c. "Don't worry, you'll feel better once you're home."
   d. "Maybe we better hold off on your discharge."

3. A patient states, "I have no reason to live. It's over." The nurse responds by saying, "It sounds like you are having thoughts about hurting yourself." In this situation, the nurse is using which of the following techniques?
   a. Confrontation
   b. Observation
   c. Reflection
   d. Interpretation
4. Which of the following behaviors when demonstrated by the nurse may interfere with communication?
   a. Direct eye contact
   b. Crossing the arms on the chest
   c. Forward leaning sitting position
   d. Sitting with both feet on the floor
5. A therapeutic relationship focuses primarily on:
   a. Patient's problems and concerns
   b. The nurse's need for information
   c. Giving advice to the patient
   d. The words used to communicate
6. In which of the following interactions does the nurse challenge the patient?
   a. Patient: "I can't sleep, its too noisy."/ Nurse: "So close your door and turn off the light."
   b. Patient: "Everyone thinks I'm evil."/ Nurse: "You're a really good person."
   c. Patient: "I'm an astronaut."/ Nurse: "So, if you're an astronaut, why aren't you on the moon?"
   d. Patient: "I'm sorry I hurt my mother."/ Nurse: "You should be. How could you hurt your mother?"
7. A patient frequently states that there are "guns going off all over the place." Whenever he states this, the nurse notices that he appears visibly anxious and scared. The patient is using which of the following to express his feelings?
   a. Symbolism
   b. Validation
   c. Empathy
   d. Rapport
8. While talking with a patient about his relationship with his deceased father, the patient tells the nurse about all the good times he had with him while fishing. "It was special. We'd talk and laugh and tell jokes." The nurse pictures the patient and his father laughing and enjoying the activity, realizing how special it was. The nurse is displaying:
   a. Self-awareness
   b. Acceptance
   c. Agreement
   d. Empathy
9. Using Peplau's model, during which phase of the nurse-patient relationship would the nurse assist the patient to develop responses to cues?
   a. Orientation
   b. Working
   c. Resolution
   d. Termination
10. When assessing one's self, which of the following would characterize the social dimension?
    a. Genetic composition
    b. Views on human nature
    c. Traits such as height
    d. Religious beliefs

Critical thinking exercises

1. Evaluate an interaction that you had with a close friend and then compare it to one that you had with a patient. How are they similar? Different?

2. Have someone videotape you and another student role-playing a nurse-patient interaction. Analyze the verbal and nonverbal communication techniques used, including body language.

3. Have your fellow students critique a process recording that you have completed. For areas identified as nontherapeutic, suggest alternative strategies to enhance your therapeutic effectiveness.

10 ▪ *The assessment process*

CHAPTER HIGHLIGHTS

Chapter 10 examines assessment as a process involving specific techniques of data collection. It explores each dimension of a biopsychosocial framework, reviewing the necessary information to be gathered.

Chapter 10 key points include the following:

- Assessment is the deliberate and systematic collection of biopsychosocial information to determine current and past health and functional status and to evaluate present and past coping patterns.
- Different types of assessment include comprehensive, screening, and ongoing assessments.
- Data collection techniques include patient observation, patient and family interviews, physical and mental examinations, records and diagnostic reports, and collaboration with colleagues.
- Biologic assessment includes present and past health status, physical examination with review of body systems, neurologic status, lab results, physical functioning, activity and exercise, sleep, appetite and nutrition, hydration, sexuality and self-care, pharmacologic assessment, and mental status examination.
- Psychological assessment includes mental status examination (general observations of appearance, psychomotor activity and attitude, orientation, mood, affection, emotion, and speech and thought processes), behavioral responses (self-concept and positive coping mechanisms), and risk factor assessment (determining suicidal assaultive or homicidal ideation).
- Social assessment includes functional status, social systems, culture, family, community and support resources, and spiritual, occupational, economic, and legal status.

STUDENT ACTIVITIES

Crossword puzzle

Across

1. Varying emotional expression
3. Attitude about one's self
5. Reaching a logical decision
6. Immediate memory
8. Thinking and knowing

Down

1. Systematic data collection
2. Awareness of one's own thoughts and feelings compared to others
4. Normal mood
7. Expressed exhibited emotion

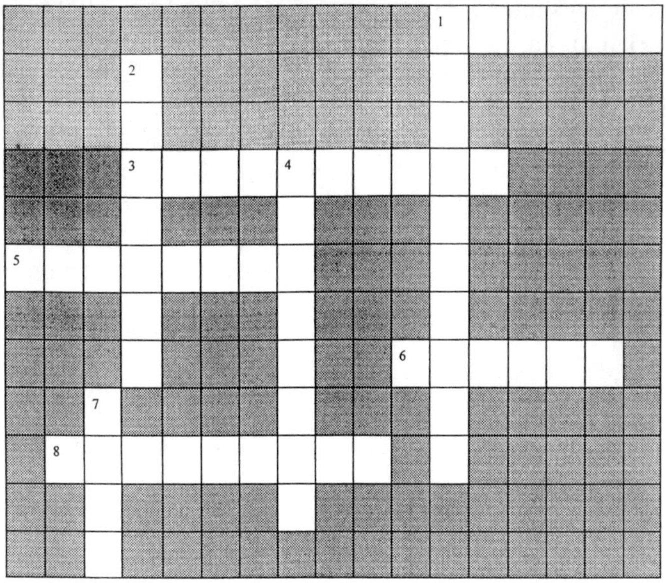

Fill in the blanks

Read each statement carefully and place your answer in the space(s) provided.

1. ________________ assessments are made to monitor the progress and outcomes of interventions implemented.
2. Usually, the basis for beginning the assessment is the ______________________________.
3. Questioning a patient about sexuality issues requires that the nurse be comfortable with one's ____.
4. The ____________ provides information about the accuracy of the patient as a reliable historian.
5. ________________ fluctuates with thought content.
6. The ________________ is a tool commonly used to assess a patient's cognition and intellectual performance.
7. Self-concept involves three interrelated dimensions: ________________, ______________, and ____.

Self-exploration

1. Answer the questions listed in text box 10-1 (in the textbook), Self Concept Awareness. Self-concept awareness to evaluate your awareness of your own self-concept. Analyze your answers to determine how your self-concept might positively or negatively impact your interactions with patients.

2. As part of a clinical assignment, your instructor asks you to draw a self-portrait and interpret your drawing based on size, color, detail, pressure, line quality, symmetry, and placement. You are to present this information for discussion in post-conference the next day. What information did you discover about yourself?

Multiple choice

Circle the option that best answers the question.

1. During assessment, the nurse demonstrates empathy by which of the following statements?
   a. "How are you feeling today?"
   b. "Where do you live?"
   c. "That must have been terrifying for you."
   d. "You feel afraid in new situations."

2. In an attempt to gather more information, the nurse plans to speak with the patient's relatives. Before doing so, the nurse must:
   a. Document the need for additional information in the chart
   b. Obtain the patient's permission to talk to them

c. Complete the physical examination
d. Notify the physician about the need for more information

3. The nurse identifies that a patient needs assistance with his current living situation. In response, the nurse would contact which member of the multidisciplinary team for assistance?
a. Social worker
b. Physical therapist
c. Psychiatrist
d. Occupational therapist

4. While talking with a patient, the nurse observes that the patient frequently shifts from anger to pleasure, crying to laughing inappropriately. When describing this patient's affect, the nurse documents it as:
a. Flat
b. Labile
c. Constricted
d. Blunted

5. A nurse asks a patient to interpret the following statement, "A penny saved is a penny earned," to assess the patient's:
a. Attention and concentration
b. Judgment and insight
c. Recall and short-term memory
d. Abstract reasoning and comprehension

6. During a patient assessment, the female patient states, "I look so horrible with this scar on my face. No guy would ever want to go out with me." On examination, the patient is wearing a scarf that covers the side of her face on which the scar is located. The scar line is pencil thin and approximately ½" long. The nurse interprets this information as a problem with the patient's:
a. Body image
b. Self-esteem
c. Self-concept
d. Personal identity

7. A patient is asked to draw a self-portrait. When analyzing the drawing, the nurse notices a lack of symmetry in the picture in how the patient placed the body parts. The nurse understands that this may represent which of the following?
a. Autonomy
b. Insecurity
c. Powerlessness
d. Confidence

8. When reviewing the complete blood count obtained for a patient receiving lithium, the nurse would expect to find which of the following?
a. Agranulocytosis
b. Polycythemia
c. Leukocytosis
d. Decreased hemoglobin

9. A patient with an eating disorder is using self-induced vomiting to purge. Which of the following laboratory results would help to support this?
a. Elevated serum potassium levels
b. Decreased platelet levels
c. Decreased serum bicarbonate levels
d. Elevated serum amylase levels

Critical thinking exercises

1. For an assigned patient in your clinical area, assess the patient's mental status using the Mini Mental State Exam, found in text box 10-5. After calculating the patient's score, identify any areas that are deficient and project possible strategies to assess these areas more closely.

2. Analyze the narrative note presented in text box 10-3 for the types of data gathered. In the chart below, classify the specific information by its type based on your synthesis of the biopsychosocial framework.

Biologic dimension	*Psychological dimension*	*Social dimension*

3. Compare and contrast the various types of formats that can be used to record assessment information, being sure to include advantages and disadvantages of each.

11 ▪ *Diagnosis and outcome development*

CHAPTER HIGHLIGHTS

Chapter 11 reviews the development of nursing diagnoses and outcomes for psychiatric mental health nursing. It examines nursing diagnosis derivation, including defining characteristics and related factors and the development, definition, purpose, and types of patient outcomes as an important component of the nursing process.

Chapter 11 key points include the following:

- With the advent of managed care, patient outcomes have become important in the evaluation of care. This is further supported by statements in the Standards for Psychiatric and Mental Health Nursing Clinical Practice.
- Outcome identification must be patient-focused and measurable. Today, more research is needed to identify patient outcomes as they related to nursing interventions.
- Assessment data provide the basis for nursing diagnoses, interventions, and patient outcomes.
- Outcome criteria can be positive or negative.
- Initial, revised, and discharge outcomes should be included in a patient's plan of nursing care.
- Outcome statements should address the biopsychosocial domains.
- Outcomes, when written properly, contain a subject, verb, circumstances, and standard of performance.

STUDENT ACTIVITIES

Short answer

Write your answer to the question in the space provided.

1. From what are nursing diagnoses developed?

2. What term is used to refer to the patient's response to care received?

3. Outcomes are the result of which step of the nursing process?

4. What are developed to direct and measure the result of nursing interventions?

5. Outcomes are the driving force for what process?

6. What four components must be included in a properly written outcome statement?

7. What are the four categories of related factors used to establish a nursing diagnosis?

Word find

Hidden within the following letter grid are key terms from chapter 11, listed below. The terms may be vertical, horizontal, diagonal, or backward. Circle the words as you find them.

Clinical path	Outcomes
Defining characteristics	Outcome criteria
Initial outcomes	Related factors
Nursing diagnosis	Standard of performance

T	C	T	I	V	E	O	S	T	U	O	C
U	R	O	U	T	C	U	O	D	S	M	E
O	I	A	R	T	D	T	M	E	D	E	C
E	T	G	E	I	E	C	M	F	O	L	N
V	E	E	H	N	F	O	T	I	I	N	A
I	R	N	A	I	C	M	O	N	M	U	M
T	S	S	B	T	I	E	I	I	A	R	R
A	E	R	U	I	N	C	P	N	I	S	O
G	M	O	L	A	A	R	R	G	N	I	F
E	O	T	I	L	G	I	A	C	C	N	R
N	C	C	P	O	D	T	C	H	S	G	E
I	T	A	T	U	I	E	T	A	T	D	P
N	T	F	A	T	S	R	I	R	N	I	F
H	A	D	T	C	C	I	C	A	A	A	O
A	R	E	I	O	H	A	A	C	E	G	D
M	I	T	O	M	R	T	I	T	M	N	R
U	A	A	N	E	G	N	L	E	E	O	A
H	H	L	P	S	I	G	A	R	T	S	D
B	K	E	M	L	S	T	Y	I	L	I	N
E	T	R	C	F	S	C	T	S	A	S	A
F	O	N	T	A	R	L	O	T	T	T	T
O	P	A	H	T	I	S	R	I	S	C	S
C	H	A	R	A	C	T	E	C	R	I	S

Multiple choice

Circle the option that best answers the question.

1. The nurse identifies the nursing diagnosis of anticipatory grieving. Which of the following statements would be an appropriate outcome?
   a. Crying lessened with hand holding
   b. Patient describes feelings of anger and helplessness
   c. Supportive feedback given to verbal concerns
   d. Risk for injury related to grief
2. The nurse is teaching a patient about the possible side effects of a new drug therapy prescribed. This action is most appropriate from which of the following?
   a. Risk for injury
   b. Ineffective individual coping
   c. Noncompliance
   d. Knowledge deficit
3. Which of the following outcomes is correctly written?
   a. The patient understands the reason for antidepressant medication
   b. The patient accepts treatment by the second day of admission
   c. The patient performs insulin self-injection correctly by the third teaching session
   d. The patient states relief of pain
4. When determining nursing diagnoses, the nurse understands that related factors:
   a. Form the foundation for the nursing diagnosis chosen
   b. Support the change in health status
   c. Are the clues given by the assessment signs and symptoms
   d. Provide information to develop outcomes

5. Outcomes are established during which step of the nursing process?
   a. Assessment
   b. Planning
   c. Implementation
   d. Evaluation
6. After determining that the outcomes the nurse previously developed were not met, the nurse writes new outcomes. These new outcomes are known as:
   a. Initial
   b. Revised
   c. Discharge
   d. Outcome criteria
7. While assessing a patient, the patient admits to having a suicide plan. In response, the nurse institutes suicide precautions based on which of the following nursing diagnoses?
   a. Powerlessness
   b. Personal identity disturbance
   c. Risk for self-directed violence
   d. Chronic low self-esteem

Critical thinking exercises

1. Review the NANDA taxonomy listing of nursing diagnoses. Categorize each nursing diagnosis as biologic, psychological, or social.

2. For each of the following nursing diagnoses listed below, develop an appropriate outcome with accompanying outcome criteria that could be used to evaluate the success of the outcome.

Nursing diagnosis	*Outcome*	*Outcome criteria*
Anxiety		
Fear		
Ineffective individual coping		
Knowledge deficit		
Self-esteem disturbance		

12 · *Biopsychosocial interventions*

CHAPTER HIGHLIGHTS

Chapter 12 explores the three major dimensions of interventions for psychiatric mental health nursing—biologic, psychological, and social. Biologic interventions focus on the physical dimensions of the individual and include self-care activities activity and exercise, nutrition, relaxation, hydration, thermoregulation, and pain and medication management. Psychological interventions address emotion, behavior, cognition, and emotion focused coping and include counseling, such as conflict resolution, bibliotherapy and reminiscence, behavior therapy, cognitive therapy, psychoeducation, health teaching, and spiritual care. Social interventions are geared to couples, families, friends, and large and small social groups with special attention to ethnicity and community interactions and include group, family, and milieu therapy, safety promotion on psychiatric units, and care delivery in the community, such as home visits and community actions.

Chapter 12 key points include the following:

- Nursing interventions, developed from assessment data and organized around nursing diagnoses, are guided by patient outcomes and *Statements on Psychiatric Mental Health Clinical Nursing* and *Standards of Psychiatric Mental Health Nursing Practice.*
- Orem's self-care deficit theory is often used to implement interventions to assist patients with psychiatric disorders to manage self-care activities.
- The nurse-patient relationship, the basic intervention of psychiatric mental health nursing, is established during implementation of other interventions.
- Medication management, a biologic intervention, is important because most persons with psychiatric disorders are prescribed medications.
- Implementation of psychobiological interventions requires a broad theoretical knowledge base.
- Psychosocial rehabilitation, closely aligned with psychoeducation, focuses on the patient's abilities, rather than the disorder and its symptoms to increase the patient's functioning within his environment. The nurse teaches, supports, and facilitates the patient's development of skills and support sources needed for successful living, learning, and working in the community.
- Group and family interventions use a system approach with a limited number of people.
- Milieu therapy, when used on an inpatient psychiatric unit, attempts to maximize the treatment effects on the patient's environment.

STUDENT ACTIVITIES

Matching

Place the letter of the description in the righthand column next to the correct item in the lefthand column.

_______ 1. Spirituality
_______ 2. Group think
_______ 3. Surveillance
_______ 4. Bibliotherpay
_______ 5. Milieu therapy
_______ 6. Reminiscence
_______ 7. Seclusion
_______ 8. Religiosity
_______ 9. Cognitive therapy
_______ 10. Group dynamics

a. Thoughts about past experiences
b. Examination of the meaning of events to change a person's view of the world
c. Excessive or affected piety
d. Provision of a stable and coherent social organization that facilitates an individual's treatment
e. Interactions within a collection of two or more persons with an interdependent relationship
f. Ongoing collection and analysis of information about a patient's environment
g. Beliefs and values related to hope and meaning of life
h. Use of selected written materials for therapeutic purposes
i. Adoption of thinking consistent with the leader's idea to avoid conflict
j. Solitary containment in a fully protective environment

Labeling

Below is a list of interventions. Place the letter of the intervention in the appropriate Nursing Intervention Classification box.

a. Using guided imagery to alleviate stress
b. Performing passive range of motion exercises to an immobile arm
c. Placing a patient in seclusion
d. Monitoring serum potassium levels for changes
e. Providing a chair for the patient to sit on while at the sink (rather than stand) to brush his teeth
f. Arranging for help with child care for the parents of a criticallzy ill infant
g. Planning a home care team conference for a newly discharged patient
h. Referring a family to a local Alzheimer's support group
i. Instructing a patient about the possible adverse effects of his antidepressant medication
j. Facilitating open communication among family members
k. Using conflict resolution in a crisis
l. Administering a medication on an empty stomach to enhance its absorption

Basic Physiologic	*Complex Physiologic*
Behavioral	*Safety*
Family	*Health System*

Fill in the blanks

Read each statement carefully and place your answer in the space(s) provided.

1. The ________________ is the core intervention of psychiatric mental health nursing.
2. ________________ is the purposeful focusing of attention away from undesirable sensations.
3. ________________ and ________________ are important in resolving any patient or family conflict.
4. Bibliotherapy can help enrich a patient's life through ____________, ________________, and ______________.
5. ______________ focuses on the strengths of the individual and also in teaching the individual how to live with the disability or problem.
6. In a ______________ group, all members begin at one time and no new members are admitted.
7. Small groups usually consist of approximately ______________ members, whereas large groups consist of ______________ members.
8. William Schutz identified three phases of group development— ________________, ________________, and ________________.
9. ________________ express the group members underlying concerns or feelings regardless of the group's purpose.
10. In a therapeutic environment, patient individuality is affirmed through ________________.

Multiple choice

Circle the letter of the option that best answers the question.

1. A salesman states that he becomes extremely anxious when he has to do a presentation in front of a group. To help him control his anxiety, the nurse instructs him to count to 20 slowly, taking a deep breath with every even number. This is an example of which relaxation technique?
   a. Simple relaxation
   b. Distraction
   c. Guided imagery
   d. Biofeedback
2. For the patient with pain, the key to effective management involves which of the following?
   a. Identifying the interaction between stress and pain
   b. Providing education about the causes of pain
   c. Identifying how the pain disrupts the person's functioning
   d. Assisting with development of cognitive skills to manage the pain
3. When attempting to resolve a conflict, the nurse should:
   a. Use her/his own view as the basis for identifying the problem
   b. Side with those individuals whose ideas seem most appropriate
   c. Develop limited solutions that meet the needs of the key individuals
   d. Help de-escalate emotion of the individuals involved in the conflict
4. An elderly Jewish patient is asked to read an article about Holocaust survivors in an attempt to elicit his feelings about his similar experience. The nurse is using which of the following techniques?
   a. Bibliotherapy
   b. Reminiscence
   c. Conflict resolution
   d. Behavior therapy
5. As the leader of a group, which of the following statements illustrates the use of clarification?
   a. "I notice that you look down and wring your hands every time the subject of sex comes up."
   b. "Could you tell us more about your relationship with your siblings?"
   c. "What I hear you saying is that you are feeling very sad now."
   d. "This is the fourth time you've changed the subject. Is something going on?"
6. Which of the following characterizes families with Pattern II relationships?
   a. Difficulty with relationships and attachment
   b. Actively seeking out professional help
   c. Overwhelming neediness with rapid attachment
   d. Functioning with intact support systems

7. When promoting patient safety on a psychiatric unit, which of the following interventions should be used as the last resort?
   a. Physical restraint
   b. Surveillance
   c. Seclusion
   d. Area restriction

8. When working with the family and caregivers, which of the following activities helps to promote family cohesion and unity?
   a. Designing schedules for activities within the family's routines
   b. Collaborating with family in problem solving and communication
   c. Teaching about health maintenance and restorative strategies
   d. Supporting adaptive family coping mechanisms

Critical thinking exercises

1. Compare and contrast the four NIC safety interventions frequently used by psychiatric nurses—surveillance, area restriction, seclusion, and chemical and physical restraint. Include specific indications and nursing actions for each.

2. Look back on a time when you experienced a conflict. Using the model shown in figure 12-2 of the text:
   a. Evaluate how this conflict was resolved.

   b. Propose an alternative yet workable resolution.

3. Visit a long-term inpatient psychiatric setting. Describe how this setting uses each of the following processes of Milieu therapy:

   Containment:

   Support:

   Validation:

   Structured Interaction:

   Open Communication:

   Arrangement of Patient Environment:

   Maintaining Ties:

4. You are assigned to teach a group of adolescent girls about eating disorders. The girls range in age from 13 to 17 years. Using the model in figure 12-4 of the text, develop an effective teaching plan that meets the needs of this audience.

13 ▪ *Nursing practice within a continuum of care*

CHAPTER HIGHLIGHTS

Chapter 13 examines the nursing practice within the continuum of care with an emphasis on the least restrictive environment. It explores the components of this continuum including inpatient care, outpatient care, managed care, and psychiatric rehabilitation, addressing the nurse's role at different points along the continuum.

Chapter 13 key points include the following:

- Continuum of care is a comprehensive system of programs and services to maintain the individual's needs with appropriate treatment in a variety of settings. These settings vary according to the level of service, structure, and intensity of care.
- The responsibilities of the psychiatric nurse vary with the setting. In most settings, they function as a member of a multidisciplinary team.
- Discharge planning provides patients with the necessary resources to function effectively in the community, thus avoiding rehospitalization.
- Managed care is influencing the continuum of care by standardizing admission criteria and clinical guidelines, encouraging use of alternative treatment programs and providing an integrated network of credentialed specialty behavioral health providers.

STUDENT ACTIVITIES

Word find

Hidden within the following letter grid are key terms from chapter 13, listed below. The terms may be horizontal, vertical, diagonal, or backward. Circle the words as you find them

Case management	Referral
Clubhouse model	Reintegration
Continuum of care	Relapse
Discharge planning	Stabilization

V	I	C	T	Y	C	M	A	N	A	G	E	K	A	R	E	D	L	N	T
M	O	D	L	E	O	L	S	T	A	B	I	L	I	Z	A	T	I	O	N
S	T	O	U	R	N	C	U	N	T	R	T	R	E	E	T	M	O	I	E
V	A	Y	Z	L	T	R	Y	B	Q	A	R	S	U	T	O	E	N	T	M
X	C	H	G	W	I	U	G	P	H	C	O	N	P	I	R	T	M	A	E
O	X	F	T	B	N	X	R	S	Z	O	W	E	V	A	C	N	O	R	G
T	E	I	T	N	U	T	A	Y	I	R	U	T	I	C	R	O	N	G	A
D	D	W	S	I	U	V	E	C	H	A	M	S	I	T	E	C	T	E	N
N	U	V	E	L	M	O	R	E	L	A	P	S	E	U	T	A	I	T	A
F	L	M	N	O	O	E	L	E	R	E	F	A	L	M	Z	Y	V	N	M
L	A	R	R	E	F	E	R	I	F	H	O	I	O	N	O	B	E	I	E
A	J	K	S	S	C	D	T	O	X	I	C	A	T	P	S	D	D	E	S
G	N	I	N	N	A	L	P	E	G	R	A	H	C	S	I	D	E	R	A
R	P	A	Q	R	R	X	O	M	L	A	S	P	R	E	R	A	L	L	C
A	R	F	O	S	E	T	R	E	R	A	C	K	O	F	T	I	A	N	N
T	O	X	I	F	I	C	A	T	I	O	N	D	E	R	E	S	I	D	E

Short answer

Write your answer to the question in the space provided.

1. Identify the time when the concept of continuum of care began.

2. Name the two methods by which one enters into the inpatient level of care.

3. Define long-term care.

4. State the most common method for providing inpatient care.

5. Identify the primary purpose of stabilization.

6. List the two major goals of in-home mental health care.

7. Name the six key principles of comprehensive in-home treatment as identified by the Bay Area Model for Psychiatric Health Care.

8. List four models of alternative housing.

9. State the goal of psychiatric rehabilitation.

10. List six domains pertinent to successful discharge of psychiatric patients.

Multiple choice

Circle the option that best answers the question.

1. A patient is involuntary committed to an inpatient facility for treatment. The primary focus of the patient's treatment is on which of the following?
   a. Educating about psychopharmacology
   b. Stabilizing acute symptoms
   c. Achieving a basic functional level
   d. Promoting independence within the community
2. A patient is scheduled for admission to a partial hospitalization program. When explaining this type of care to the patient and his family, the nurse is correct when stating that this type of program:
   a. Does not provide overnight care
   b. Provides little recreational activities
   c. Runs seven days a week
   d. Offers limited behavioral interventions
3. Assessment of a patient reveals moderate to severe symptoms of an exacerbation of a persistent mental disorder with marked impairment in his ADLs of nutrition and hygiene. This patient would be appropriate for which of the following levels of ambulatory care?
   a. Level I
   b. Level II
   c. Level III
   d. None
4. Which of the following statements best describes the nurse's role as a generalist case manager?
   a. Direct service provider within the agency
   b. Management of symptoms
   c. Coordination of care with multiple agencies
   d. Administration of psychopharmacologic agents
5. A patient with a mental disorder has returned to work but still requires routine psychiatric services for stabilization. Which of the following programs would be the most likely choice?
   a. Intensive outpatient program
   b. Personal care home
   c. Therapeutic foster care
   d. Clubhouse
6. Determining the level of care necessary for a patient who is to receive psychiatric rehabilitation is based on which of the following?
   a. DSM IV diagnosis
   b. Financial resources available
   c. Projected treatment plan
   d. Need identification and matching
7. A patient is to receive Level I ambulatory behavioral care. Which of the following settings would be appropriate?
   a. Clubhouse program
   b. Assertive community treatment
   c. Psychosocial rehabilitation
   d. Partial hospitalization
8. A patient is referred for in-home detoxification. In planning for this patient's care, the nurse anticipates that during the first week of sobriety, visits need to be made:
   a. Daily
   b. Twice a day
   c. Every other day
   d. Twice a week

Critical thinking exercises

1. Using an assigned patient from your clinical experience and the Mental Health Discharge checklist form (text box 13-2, in the textbook), prepare a discharge plan for the patient that addresses his biopsychosocial needs, discharge interventions, and aftercare.

2. Imagine that you are assigned to teach a group of nursing students about the continuum of care for mental health. Create a diagram that you can use in your presentation to illustrate the various components along the continuum.

3. Interview a nurse who works as a case manager in psychiatric mental health. Identify the roles this person assumes and provide examples of the activities performed in each of these roles.

4. Investigate a psychiatric rehabilitation program in your area and evaluate the schedules used for specific mental health and psychiatric disorders.

UNIT FOUR
Care of persons with psychiatric disorders

14 ▪ *Schizophrenia*

CHAPTER HIGHLIGHTS

Chapter 14 explores the clinically complex psychiatric disorder of schizophrenia through integration of the biopsychosocial framework. It reviews the definition, diagnostic criteria, and epidemiologic aspects of the disorder including distribution, ethnic, cultural, and gender differences, age at onset, comorbidity, and risk factors and addresses possible etiologic theories and somatic interventions. Applying the nursing process, this chapter describes the nursing management of a patient diagnosed with schizophrenia.

Chapter 14 key points include the following:

- Schizophrenia involves a complex myriad of positive and negative symptoms. Positive symptoms, those that exist but should not, include delusions or hallucinations and disorganized thinking and behavior. Negative symptoms, those characteristics that should be present but are lacking, include alogia, avolition, anhedonia, and affective blunting.
- Previously, diagnosis and treatment have focused on more observable and dramatic positive symptoms. Recently, focus has shifted to the disorganizing symptoms of cognition.
- Schizophrenia clinically presents three phases—Phase I (initial diagnosis and first treatment); Phase II (period of relative calm between episodes of overt signs and symptoms but during which the patient needs sustained treatment); and Phase III (periods of exacerbation or relapse requiring hospitalization or more frequent contact with mental health professional and increased use of resources).
- Schizophrenia, found in approximately 1 in 10,000 people and most commonly diagnosed in late adolescence and early adulthood, is clustered in lowest classes in industrialized urban communities.
- Biologic theories of causation include genetic, infectious-autoimmune, neuroanatomic, theories and dopamine hypothesis (supported by advanced technology of PET scan findings and understanding of antipsychotic agents' mechanism of action).
- Antipsychotic agents, which generally block dopamine transmission in the brain, are associated with troublesome and sometimes serious anticholinergic and extrapyramidal side effects. Nurses need to be familiar with these agents, their side effects, and interventions necessary to manage or control them.
- Extrapyramidal side effects including acute Parkinsonism, pseudo Parkinsonism, acute dystonia, and akathisia, can appear early or late (months to years) during treatment. Tardive dyskinesia, a late appearing extrapyramidal side effect, is a severe syndrome of abnormal motor movements of the mouth, tongue, and jaw.
- Biologic assessment must include a thorough history and physical examination to rule out any possible medical illness or substance abuse problems as the cause, assessment of risk of injury to self or others, and creation of baseline health information before medications are begun.

- Psychological assessment must include equal attention to manifestations of both positive and negative symptoms and a concentrated focus on cognitive impairments that make it so difficult for these patients to manage their disorder.
- Standardized assessment tools are available to assess characteristic abnormal motor movements and positive and negative symptoms.
- Primary interventions include psychopharmacology in conjunction with cognitive therapy to assist with coping and adjustment to the disorder.
- Schizophrenia is a lifetime disorder that requires continued support and care from mental health professionals and family or friends. Education about the course of the disorder, importance of drug maintenance, and the need for consistent care and support is one primary nursing intervention.
- Research is demonstrating that interactions between patients and their families is key to the success of long-term treatment and outcomes.

STUDENT ACTIVITIES

Matching

Place the letter of the description from the righthand column next to the correct term in the left-hand column.

_______ 1. Anhedonia
_______ 2. Hallucinations
_______ 3. Circumstantiality
_______ 4. Neologisms
_______ 5. Verbigeration
_______ 6. Illusions
_______ 7. Echopraxia
_______ 8. Akathisia
_______ 9. Avolition
_______ 10. Echolalia

a. Made up words with no common meaning and not recognizable
b. Misperceptions or exaggeration of actual stimuli in the environment
c. Involuntary imitation of another person's movement and gestures
d. Motor restlessness
e. Inability to experience pleasure
f. Parrotlike and inappropriate repetition of another's words
g. Perceptual experiences occurring in absence of external sensory stimuli
h. Withdrawal and inability to initiate and persist in goal-directed activity
i. Extremely lengthy discourse about a topic
j. Purposeless repetition of words or phrases

Short answer

Write your answer to the question in the space provided.

1. For each item listed below, identify whether it is a positive or negative symptom of schizophrenia:
   a. Grandiose delusions

   b. Flat affect

   c. Loose associations

   d. Alogia

   e. Autistic thinking

f. Hypervigilance

g. Echopraxia

h. Anhedonia

2. For each characteristic listed below, identify the phase during which it would most likely occur:
   a. Lack of overt symptoms

   b. First diagnosis

   c. Hospitalization for exacerbation

   d. Increased use of community resources for relapse

   e. Stabilization of symptoms with therapy

3. Based on the average age of first episode, name the sex in which schizophrenia is diagnosed earlier.

4. List two other disorders commonly seen in patients with schizophrenia.

5. Identify the three changes in brain structure that have been found in patients who have had schizophrenia.

6. Name the site in the brain believed to be involved with the extrapyramidal side effects of antipsychotic drugs.

7. State the presenting symptoms of neuroleptic malignant syndrome (NMS).

8. List the three phases of antipsychotic medication treatment.

9. Name two possible indications for using ECT with patients with schizophrenia.

10. Identify the most frequent type of hallucination seen with schizophrenia.

Multiple choice

Circle the option that best answers the question.

1. During an interview with a patient diagnosed with schizophrenia, the nurse asks, "How are you feeling?" The patient responds by saying, "Feeling, reeling, stealing, kneeling." The nurse interprets this response as which of the following?
   a. Echolalia
   b. Neologism
   c. Clang association
   d. Flight of ideas
2. When planning a teaching session about the epidemiology of schizophrenia for a group of families with a member diagnosed with this disorder, the nurse incorporates which of the following concepts into the teaching plan?
   a. Schizophrenia is more prevalent in high social economic classes
   b. Schizophrenia is most commonly diagnosed in late adolescence and early adulthood
   c. Men are more commonly diagnosed with schizophrenia than women
   d. Auditory hallucinations are more common in younger patients diagnosed with schizophrenia
3. During assessment, a patient states, "I am omnipotent. I control the world and all of its money. No one can hurt me." The nurse determines that this patient is experiencing delusions and is correct in documenting them as which of the following?
   a. Grandiose
   b. Nihilistic
   c. Persecutory
   d. Somatic
4. When administering antipsychotic agents, the nurse understands that these drugs act primarily by blocking which of the following?
   a. Acetylcholine activity
   b. Serotonin reuptake
   c. Histamine receptors
   d. Postsynaptic dopamine
5. When studying for an examination, a student is reviewing the various theories of causation for schizophrenia. The student demonstrates evidence of understanding the psychological theories by identifying which of the following as the underlying belief?
   a. Family pattern interaction
   b. Dysfunctional parenting in early childhood
   c. Genetic transmission for the disorder
   d. Infant over satisfaction during the oral stage
6. A patient is prescribed clozapine 300 mg/day. Prior to initiating therapy, the nurse anticipates the need for which of the following laboratory tests?
   a. White blood cell count
   b. Hemoglobin and hematocrit
   c. Liver functions studies
   d. Chest X ray
7. A patient experiences galactorrhea as a side effect of antipsychotic therapy. The nurse understands that this side effect is the result of the drug affecting which of the following dopaminergic tracts?
   a. Mesocortical
   b. Nigrostriatal
   c. Tuberoinfundibular
   d. Mesolimbic
8. When assessing a patient with schizophrenia, the nurse observed the patient to be laughing while talking about the death of his mother. The nurse correctly documents the patient's affect as which of the following?
   a. Flat
   b. Inappropriate
   c. Blunted
   d. Full range
9. When dealing with a patient who is experiencing hallucinations, which of the following behaviors by the nurse would not be therapeutic?
   a. Directly confronting the patient about the hallucinations
   b. Ignoring the patient's behavior
   c. Validating the observations by questioning the patient
   d. Telling the patient to pay attention

10. When teaching a patient and family about schizophrenia, the nurse stresses which of the following as the most important?
    a. Life management skills
    b. Schizophrenia as a lifetime disorder
    c. Community resources
    d. Compliance with medication therapy
11. A patient exhibits constant lip smacking and puckering, foot tapping and tongue protruding. The nurse interprets these signs as indicative of which of the following?
    a. Parkinsonism
    b. Dystonia
    c. Tardive dyskinesia
    d. Akathisia
12. A patient with schizophrenia is having difficulty maintaining his personal hygiene. As part of his plan of care, the nurse should do which of the following?
    a. Allow the patient to do whatever care he can regardless of his appearance
    b. Perform complete hygiene care, allowing him to participate in one task each day
    c. Tell the patient when it is time to get washed and dressed
    d. Break the task into a small series of steps and write it down for him

Critical thinking exercises

1. A 45-year-old patient is prescribed thioridazine (Mellaril), 150 mg P.O. t.i.d., as maintenance therapy after discharge to his parents' home. His parents are in their early seventies. The patient's father has some diminished hearing in his left ear and the patient's mother has some joint immobility in her hands and wrists related to osteoarthritis. Both parents are alert and oriented and voice a desire to care for their son. Two siblings live within close driving distance to the parents' home. Develop an appropriate teaching plan for this patient and his family, taking into consideration any limitations that the patient's caregivers might have.

2. A patient comes to the emergency department with a fever of 102 degrees F for the last 24 hours without any complaints of signs and symptoms of an infection. Physical examination reveals slight tachycardia and tachypnea, and moderate muscle rigidity of the arms. Laboratory evidence is within normal limits except for a moderate leukocytosis and elevated creatinine phosphokinase. History reveals diagnosis of schizophrenia and treatment with antipsychotic agents for the past three years. A diagnosis of neuroleptic malignant syndrome is made. After integrating your knowledge about NMS and analysis of this situation, construct an appropriate plan of care for this patient.

3. Using the patient scenario in Nursing Care Plan 14-1 (in the textbook) for Jonah and the chart below, analyze the situation for possible biopsychosocial etiologies and develop appropriate biopsychosocial outcomes and interventions.

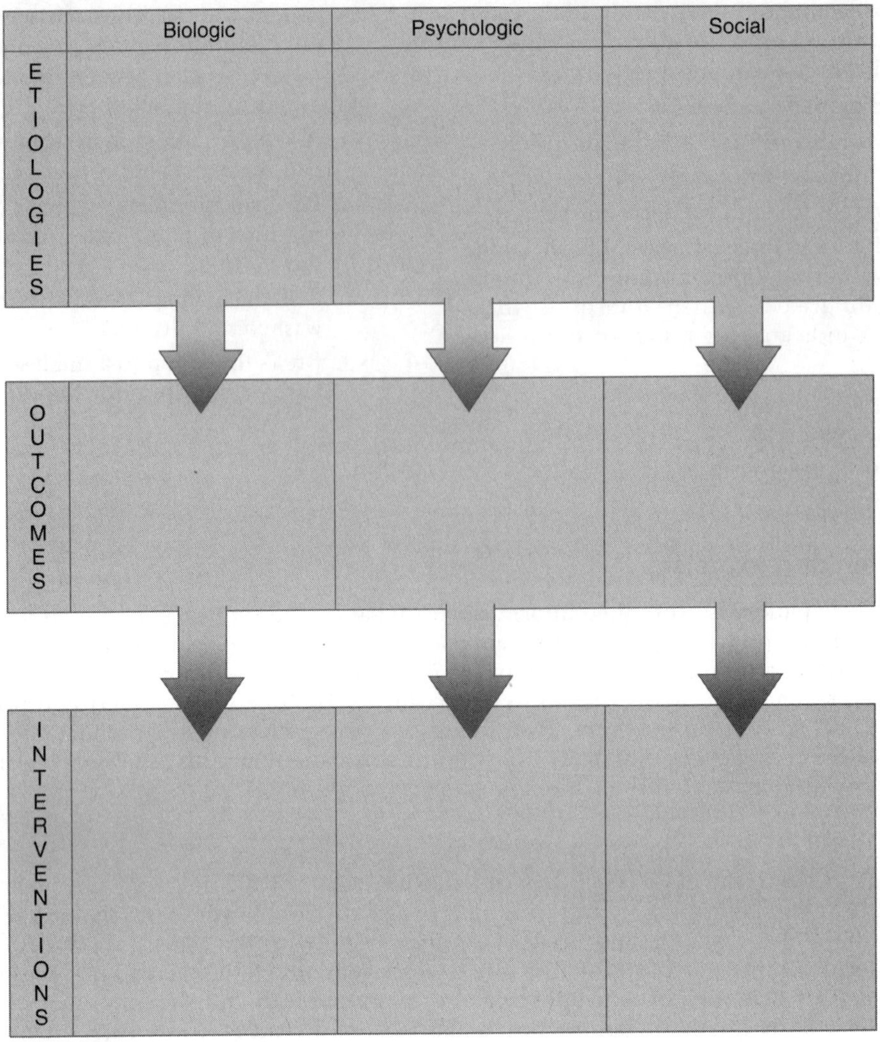

4. Compare and contrast the following antipsychotic agents, including drug class, mechanism of action, side effects, contraindications and precautions, nursing implications and patient education.

   Chlorpromazine (Thorazine)

   Mesoridazine (Serentil)

   Fluphenazine (Prolixin)

   Haloperidol (Haldol)

   Thiothixene (Navane)

   Olanzapine (Zyprexia)

5. Using the deficits listed in text box 14-3 (deficits that cause vulnerability in schizophrenia) (in the textbook), propose effective nursing interventions that would be helpful in overcoming these deficits.

15 ▪ *Schizoaffective, delusional, and other psychotic disorders*

CHAPTER HIGHLIGHTS

Chapter 15 explores other psychiatric disorders involving psychosis, such as schizophreniform, schizoaffective, delusional, brief psychotic and shared psychotic disorders. Focusing primarily on two disorders, schizoaffective and delusional disorders, it reviews the definition and epidemiologic aspects of each including distribution, age at onset, gender, ethnic, cultural, and familial differences, and comorbidity, and addresses possible etiologic theories of causation and somatic interventions. Applying the nursing process with integration of the biopsychosocial framework, the chapter describes the nursing management of a patient diagnosed with a schizoaffective or delusional disorder.

Chapter 15 key points include the following:

- Patients with schizoaffective disorder experience more problems most of the time along with positive symptoms such as delusions or hallucinations without mood symptoms at some time during the uninterrupted period of illness.
- The DSM IV identifies schizoaffective disorder as a separate category.
- Patients with schizoaffective disorder experience less awareness deficits and appear to have more insight than patients with true schizophrenia. This is helpful in teaching patients to control symptoms, recognize early regression, and develop some psychosocial skills.
- Patients with schizoaffective disorder are unlikely to be ever medication-free.
- Nursing care focuses on minimizing psychiatric symptoms by promoting medication maintenance and helping patients maintain optimal levels of functioning. Interventions focus on developing social and coping skills. Nurses need to be constantly attuned to the patient's mood, helping them learn problem solving, conflict resolution, and social situation coping.
- Delusional disorder is characterized by stable, well-systematized, and logical nonbizarre delusions that could occur in real life and are plausible within the context of the patient's ethnic and cultural background. These delusions may or may not interfere with the person's ability to function socially.
- Patients with delusional disorder typically deny any psychiatric basis for their problems and refuse to seek psychiatric care, often being seen on medical surgical units of hospitals where their delusions relate to various somatic complaints.
- Diagnosis of delusional disorder is often made only when the delusions relate to their health or when they act on the basis of their delusions and violate the law or social rules.
- Delusional disorder subtypes, classified by the nature and content of the patient's delusions include erotomanic, grandiose, jealous, somatic, mixed, and unspecified.
- Patients with delusional disorder usually do not experience any functional difficulties or mental status impairments. Their thinking, orientation, affect, attention, memory, perceptions, and personality generally remain intact.
- Establishment of a therapeutic relationship is crucial to successful treatment of delusional disorder.
- Nurses must be aware of the patient's fragile self-esteem and unusual sensitivities and anxieties and try to establish a trusting relationship through a flexible, nonjudgmental approach that promotes empathy, trust, and support, while keeping a physical and emotional detachment.

STUDENT ACTIVITIES

Word unscramble

Below is a list of scrambled words. Unscramble each word and place it in the appropriate space next to its definition.

romiaetoan   hsospycsi

islsonude   motlpticehy

isinticamdefition

_____________ 1. A state in which an individual is experiencing hallucinations, delusions, and disorganized thoughts, speech, or behavior.

_____________ 2. Effect of stabilizing one's mood.

_____________ 3. False, fixed unbreakable beliefs that fall outside the patient's social, cultural, or religious background.

_____________ 4. Belief that a person is loved intensely by a loved object who is usually married and of higher socioeconomic status, making the person unattainable.

_____________ 5. Familiar person is replaced by an imposter; illusion of doubles.

Fill in the blanks

Place the correct answer in the space(s) provided.

1. The most common type of schizoaffective disorder is _______________.
2. On MRI, patients with schizoaffective disorder have been shown to exhibit ___________ brain size and _______________.
3. The prevailing neurochemical hypothesis for schizoaffective disorder involves overactivity of _______________.
4. Approximately ¼ of patients diagnosed with schizoaffective disorder will experience _____________, for which a benzodiazepine may be prescribed.
5. _____________ is an alternative adjunctive medication that may be given to stabilize the patient's mood.
6. Hospitalization may be required at the time of an acute psychotic episode to protect the patient from _______________.
7. Patients with delusional disorder typically function at a ___________ level.
8. Hallucinations, if present with delusional disorder, typically are ___________, _____________, or __________ in nature.
9. The central theme of somatic delusions involves _______________.
10. Generally, delusional disorder occurs in _______________.

Multiple choice

Circle the option that best answers the question.

1. A patient states, "There are bugs crawling under my skin and inside my stomach. Look, look how itchy I am. I'm scratching so much." The nurse interprets this as indicative of which of the following?
   a. Grandiose delusions
   b. Somatic delusions
   c. Jealous delusions
   d. Persecutory delusions

2. When describing schizoaffective disorder to a group of nursing students, the instructor is correct in stating which of the following?
   a. Episodes are consistent with mood disorders occurring concomitantly with symptoms of schizophrenia
   b. When symptoms are intense, psychosocial functioning is still maintained
   c. Positive symptoms occur without the mood symptoms being present
   d. The depressive type appears more commonly than the bipolar type

3. Combination psychopharmacologic therapy in treatment for schizoaffective disorder has been found to be:
   a. Often effective but the response is incomplete
   b. Associated with fewer side effects and increased compliance
   c. Helpful in resolving the psychosis
   d. Necessary to reduce the dosage amount of antipsychotic agent used
4. Drug therapy is ordered for a patient with schizoaffective disorder. Which of the following drugs would the nurse expect to administer for both its mood stabilizing and antipsychotic effects?
   a. Clozapine
   b. Risperidone
   c. Valproate
   d. Lithium
5. Evaluating a patient for possible stressors is important during assessment of the patient suspected with schizoaffective disorder for which of the following reasons?
   a. Stressors affect the patient's level of self-care
   b. Knowledge of stressors uncovers the cause for the behavior
   c. Presence of stressors enhances reality contact
   d. Stressors may trigger or precipitate symptoms
6. A patient is suspected of having delusional disorder. During assessment, which of the following characteristics would the nurse determine to be indicative of this disorder?
   a. Level of intellectual function is severely impaired
   b. Numerous somatic complaints cause the patient to seek out help
   c. The patient is openly aware of the delusions
   d. Hallucinations, if present, are usually auditory in nature
7. When intervening with a patient diagnosed with delusional disorder, nursing care focuses on which of the following?
   a. Firm, limited approach
   b. Insight-oriented therapy
   c. Trusting therapeutic relationship
   d. Physical isolation and seclusion

Critical thinking exercises

1. Using the patient scenario in Nursing Care Plan 15-1 (in the textbook), Ms. K., and the chart below, analyze the situation for possible biopsychosocial etiologies and develop appropriate biopsychosocial outcomes and interventions.

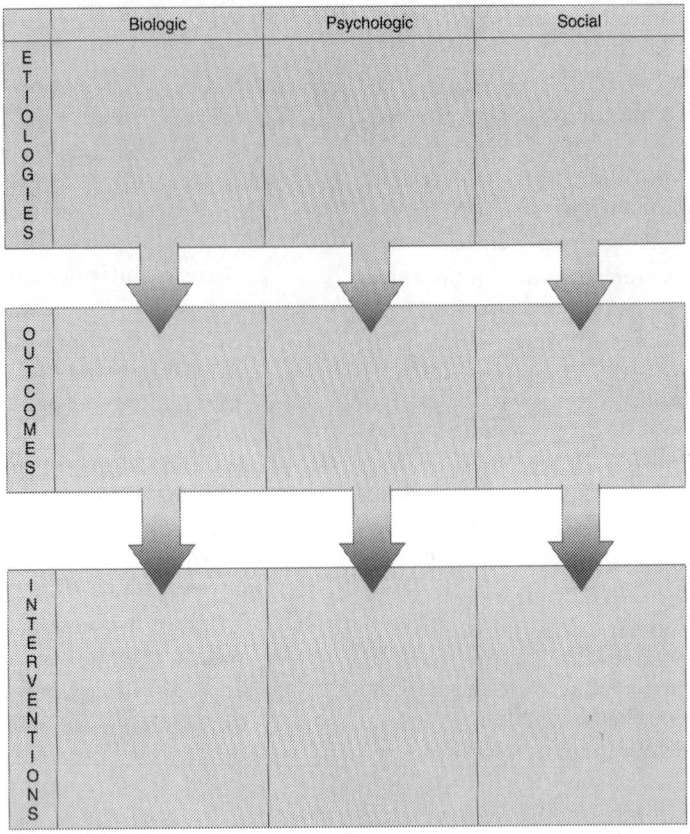

2. The following nursing diagnoses have been identified on the plan of care for a patient diagnosed with schizoaffective disorder. For each nursing diagnosis, identify possible defining characteristics and propose appropriate outcomes.

Nursing diagnosis	*Defining characteristics*	*Outcomes*
Chronic low self-esteem		
Ineffective individual coping		
Anxiety		
Altered thought process		
Social isolation		

3. Review old newspapers and magazine articles for the story about John Hinkley, Jr., his assassination attempt on President Reagan, and his relationship with actress Jodie Foster. Analyze the information and describe whether he exhibited any characteristics of delusional disorder. Support your analysis with specific examples.

16 ▪ *Mood disorders*

CHAPTER HIGHLIGHTS

Chapter 16 examines the two major mood disorders, major depressive disorder and bipolar disorders through integration of the biopsychosocial framework. It reviews the epidemiology, including distribution, age of onset, gender, ethnic, and cultural differences, comorbidity, and clinical course and addresses possible etiologic theories of causation and somatic interventions. Applying the nursing process, the chapter describes the nursing management of a patient diagnosed with either of these two disorders.

Chapter 16 key points include the following:

- Mood disorders are characterized by persistent or recurring disturbances or alterations in mood or emotion that cause significant psychological stress and behavioral impairment.
- Mood is broadly categorized as manic or euphoric (exaggerated feelings of well being or elation) or as depressive or dysphoric (extreme feelings of sadness, hopelessness, loss of interest, and fatigue).
- Primary mood disorders include depressive disorders or manic depressive disorders, characterized by the occurrence of at least one manic episode.
- A major depressive disorder, which affects all age groups and both sexes, is twice as common in adolescents and young women, with increasing rates in younger adults, adolescents, and adults over age 65.
- Genetic influences have been demonstrated as playing a substantial role in etiology of mood disorders. Other psychosocial risk factors include a family history of mood disorders, prior episodes of depression, lack of social support, stressful life events, substance abuse and medical problems, especially chronic or terminal illness.
- Recommended guidelines for treatment of depression include antidepressant medications in conjunction with psychotherapeutic management or psychotherapy.
- ECT has been used successfully for treatment of severe depression. Phototherapy has been successful in treating patients with seasonal depressive symptoms.
- Nursing knowledge about antidepressant medications is necessary for patient education and evaluation for therapeutic effectiveness. Familiarity with ECT protocols and interventions is essential for patient and family education and provision of emotional support before and during ECT.
- Because many symptoms of depression are similar to those associated with other medical problems, a thorough biologic assessment is required to rule out other medical causes.
- Psychosocial assessment areas include mood, thought processes, and psychiatric thought content, suicidal or homicidal thoughts, cognition and memory, and social factors such as family psychiatric history, changes in occupational functioning, relationship patterns, and quality of support systems.
- A therapeutic nurse-patient relationship is key for patients with major depressive disorder. Interventions include being available in times of crisis, providing understanding and education to patients and families about treatment goals, providing encouragement and feedback about the patient's progress, providing guidance in the patient's interpersonal interactions with others and the work environment, and helping to set and monitor realistic goals.
- Self-care management, cognitive, behavioral, and interpersonal therapies, patient and family education, marital and family therapy, and group therapy, including medication maintenance and other consumer-oriented support groups are appropriate psychosocial interventions.

- Bipolar disorders are characterized by one or more manic episodes or mixed mania causing marked impairment in social activities, occupational functioning and interpersonal relations. Hospitalization may be necessary to prevent self-harm.
- Manic episodes, periods in which the individual experiences abnormal and persistent elevated, expansive or irritable mood, are characterized by inflated self-esteem, decreased need to sleep, excessive energy or hyperactivity, racing thoughts, easy distractibility, and inability to stay focused. Hypersexuality and impulsivity also may be present.
- Manic states, although assumed to be pleasant experiences, are most uncomfortable, possibly resulting in serious interpersonal and occupational problems.
- Pharmacotherapy, including mood stabilizers alone or in combination with antipsychotic agents or benzodiazepines (if agitation or insomnia is present), is the cornerstone of treatment for bipolar disorders.
- ECT is a treatment alternative for severely manic patients exhibiting unremitting, frenzied physical activity.
- Psychosocial interventions and therapy are used in conjunction with pharmacotherapy. The use of integrated psychosocial and pharmacologic treatment involving family or marital based therapies and psychoeducational programs has been shown to be effective.

STUDENT ACTIVITIES

Labeling

1. For each concept listed below, determine the causative theory to which it belongs. Then place the corresponding letter in the appropriate circle on the biopsychosocial figure.
   a. Early deprivation of love and affection
   b. Lack of adequate emotional parenting
   c. Substantial adverse life event
   d. Genetic vulnerability
   e. Family problems as ongoing stressors
   f. Irrational beliefs and distorted attitudes toward self
   g. Alteration in hypothalamic-pituitary-adrenal axis
   h. Loss of an important role in life
   i Interactions among the homeostatic and regulatory functions

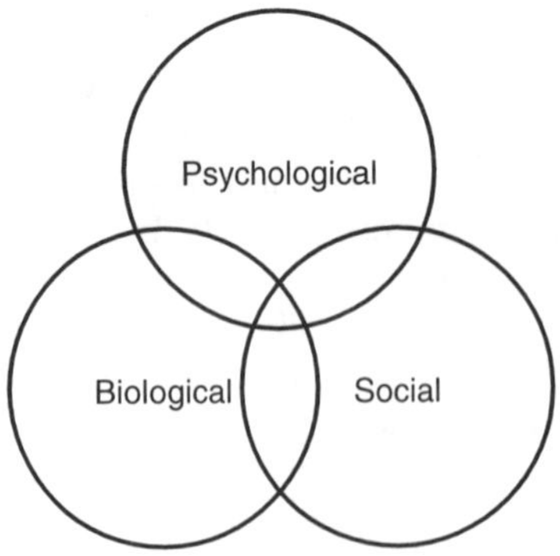

2. On the chart below, place the corresponding letter of the drug in the appropriate column.
   a. Fluoxetine (Prozac)
   b. Doxepin (Sinequan)
   c. Phenelzine (Nardil)
   d. Amitriptyline (Elavil)
   e. Paroxetine (Paxil)
   f. Buproprion (Wellbutrin)
   g. Tranylcypromine (Parnate)
   h. Mirtazapine (Remeron)

Tricyclics	*SSRIs*	*MAOIs*	*Other atypical*

Word find

Hidden within the following letter grid are key terms from chapter 16, listed below. The terms may be vertical, horizontal, diagonal, or backward. Circle the words as you find them.

Affect
Bipolar
Dysphoria
Elevated mood
Euphoria
Expansive mood
Hypomania
Lability
Mania
Manic episode
Mood
Pseudodementia
Rapid cycling
Unipolar

```
E L E C T D L R O C O N V U E L S I
E U P H O T A S E R O T O N L I N G
R A L O P I B P Y L A B I L E T Y N
A R M R D Y I A A N R E H T V E V I
L P A I E H L I P O D O R M A P X L
O E N A A A I R O H P U E I T O R C
P S I A F H T O T A Y G R X E L D Y
I S C F N A Y H R I L I N O D A I C
N I E T I E X P A N S I V E M O O D
U C P H A S E S O A I P E D O M S I
T O I E P O Y Y P M Y P I E O I E P
R N S Y R A P D I O A C D R D S O A
D Y O I N T E R D R P N X P A N R R
M H D S S O N A L E E R I A B V D O
P S E U D O D E M E N T I A S R E R
```

Multiple choice

Circle the option that best answers the question.

1. When administering antidepressant drugs, the nurse is alert for serotonin syndrome, which results from which of the following drugs?
   a. Phenelzine (Nardil)
   b. Buproprion (Wellbutrin)
   c. Fluoxetine (Prozac)
   d. Mirtazapine (Remeron)

2. When administering MAOIs to a patient, the nurse should do which of the following?
   a. Administer the drug once a day
   b. Encourage intake of raisins and bananas
   c. Administer SSRI concomitantly
   d. Monitor for possible hypertensive crisis

3. A patient who was prescribed SSRI states that he stopped taking the medication. In determining the patient's rationale for doing so, the nurse understands that the most common reason is due to which of the following?
   a. Persistent nausea
   b. Loss of sexual function
   c. Drowsiness and sedation
   d. Heart palpitations
4. When preparing a patient for ECT, the nurse informs the patient of the possibility of which of the following?
   a. Memory loss
   b. Suicidal thoughts
   c. Recurrent seizures
   d. Prolonged hypertension
5. Which of the following statements by the patient indicates effective teaching about using phototherapy for treatment of seasonal depressive symptoms?
   a. "I'll start the therapy after eating breakfast every morning, usually around 9 A.M."
   b. "I won't expect any effects for at least two weeks after I start the therapy."
   c. "I'll use the lights for approximately two hours initially, and then gradually shorten the time after one week."
   d. "Once I feel better, I'll use the lights for approximately 30 minutes each day."
6. When communicating with a patient who is depressed, which of the following approaches would most likely be ineffective?
   a. Warm and empathetic
   b. Slow and patient
   c. Enthusiastic and cheering on
   d. Guiding and encouraging
7. A patient complains of nausea secondary to antidepressant therapy. Which of the following instructions would be most helpful?
   a. Advise the patient to use sugarless gum or candies
   b. Encourage a diet rich in fresh fruits and vegetables
   c. Warn the patient to change his position slowly
   d. Suggest the patient take the drug with food
8. When teaching a family support group for bipolar disorders, the nurse is correct in stating which of the following?
   a. Manic episodes develop more abruptly than depressive episodes
   b. The manic episode is a pleasant experience for the patient
   c. With either episode, occupational functioning is usually heightened
   d. Bipolar disorders are usually acute, one time occurrences
9. A patient admitted to the psychiatric unit is diagnosed with bipolar I disorder. He requires rapid stabilization to control the severity of his symptoms. The nurse anticipate administering which of the following?
   a. Lithium (Eskalith)
   b. Divalproex sodium (Depakote)
   c. Carbamazepine (Tegretol)
   d. Haloperidol (Haldol)
10. A patient diagnosed with bipolar I disorder is prescribed lithium. The patient also has a history of hypertension for which he is receiving captopril (Capoten). Which of the following interventions would be most appropriate?
    a. Monitoring renal function studies
    b. Assessing for increased signs and symptoms of bipolar disorder
    c. Anticipating the need for increasing the dosage of lithium
    d. Anticipating the need for increasing the dosage of captopril
11. A patient diagnosed with bipolar I disorder is experiencing rapid cycling and is admitted to the inpatient psychiatric unit with psychotic symptoms and severe mania. The nurse determines that the priority nursing diagnosis for this patient would be:
    a. Sleep pattern disturbance
    b. Altered role performance
    c. Risk for injury to self
    d. Ineffective individual coping
12. Which of the following statements by a patient diagnosed with bipolar disorder on lithium therapy indicates effective teaching?
    a. "I'll call the doctor immediately if I start urinating more."
    b. "I'll increase my salt intake if it becomes hot and I start to perspire a lot."
    c. "I'll know to expect some ringing in my ears and blurred vision in the beginning."
    d. "I'll take my lithium before I eat if I experience diarrhea."

Critical thinking exercises

1. Review the therapeutic dialogue box (UNBOXTD16-1), Mr. Jones (in the textbook).
   a. Using the second scenario (effective approach), continue the interaction with him to elicit further information about the patient's feelings.

   b. Develop a plan of care that addresses this patient's priority needs.

2. Analyze the clinical vignette, found in text box 16-1 (in the textbook), about Mr. Russo to determine whether the patient meets the key diagnostic characteristics for major depressive or bipolar disorder.

3. Using the patient scenario presented in Nursing Care Plan 16-1 (in the textbook), Ms. Rothman, and the chart below, synthesize possible biopsychosocial etiologies for this patient from your analysis and develop appropriate biopsychosocial outcomes and interventions.

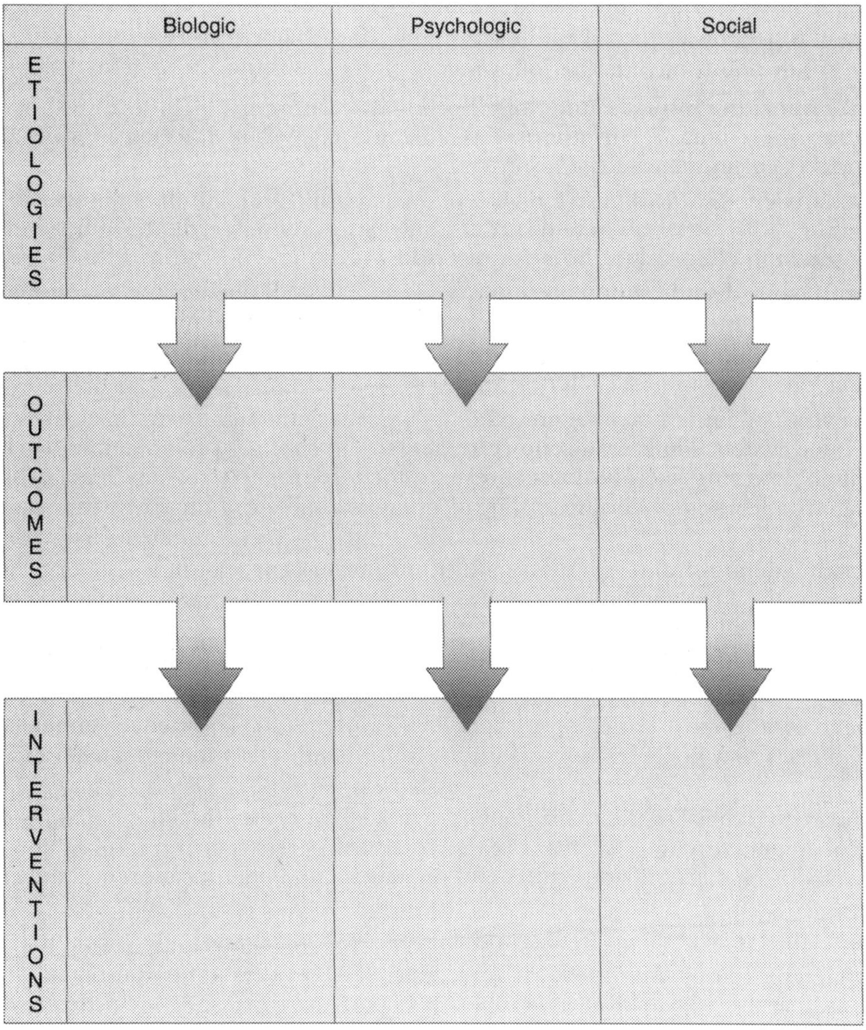

4. As part of a class assignment, an instructor asks you to think back on a time when you have said or thought that you were "depressed." Explore the biologic, psychologic, and social manifestations that you experienced.

17 ▪ *Anxiety and related disorders*

CHAPTER HIGHLIGHTS

Chapter 17 focuses on three major anxiety disorders—panic, generalized anxiety, and obsessive-compulsive disorders—and explores related disorders, such as phobia, posttraumatic stress disorder, and dissociative disorder. It reviews the epidemiology, etiology, somatic interventions, including psychopharmacology, and risk factors as appropriate for each of the three disorders. Applying the nursing process with integration of the biopsychosocial framework, the chapter describes the nursing management of a patient diagnosed with each of the three major anxiety disorders.

Chapter 17 key points include the following:

- Anxiety disorders, the most common of all psychiatric disorders, include a wide range of disorders, sharing the common symptoms of recurring anxiety but differing in symptom profiles. Panic attacks occur in many of the disorders.
- Those with anxiety disorders have a high level of physical and emotional illness, often suffering dual diagnoses with other anxiety disorders, substance abuse, or depression, rendering them unable to function effectively at home or at work.
- Patients with panic disorder often present a confusing array of physical and emotional symptoms. Skillful assessment is required to first eliminate possible life-threatening causes.
- A combination of biologic and psychosocial factors have been implicated in causing persistent anxiety.
- The initial stage of panic attack seems to be biologically generated by neural activity in the brain stem. Biologic evidence links anticipatory anxiety to the kindling phenomenon occurring in the limbic system, lowering one's biologic threshold for response to stressors. The last stage of phobic avoidance, a learned phenomenon, involves considerable cognitive activity, occurring in the prefrontal cortex.
- Other research demonstrates that personality traits, such as low self-esteem, external locus of control, some negative family influences, and some traumatic or stressful precipitating event(s) predispose an individual to anxiety disorders.
- Treatment approaches include pharmacotherapy, psychological treatment, or often a combination of both.
- Nurses need to approach patients with anxiety disorders with knowledge, understanding, and calmness. Nurses play key roles in crisis intervention, medication management, and psychoeducation.
- Psychoeducation, crucial to the management of anxiety disorders, include measures to cope with and control anxiety reactions, such as breathing control, stress reduction, relaxation techniques, education about medication side effects and management, and education of family members to understand these disorders.
- OCD, although rare, is difficult to diagnose because patients do not often seek help.
- OCD is characterized by unwanted, intrusive, and persistent thoughts causing so much anxiety and distress, that the individual feels compelled to perform ritualistic, repetitive action to reduce the agonizing anxiety.

STUDENT ACTIVITIES

Crossword puzzle

Across

1. Uncomfortable feeling of apprehension
2. Overwhelming anxiety
4. Repetitive anxiety-producing impulses
6. Generic Tofranil
7. First drug used for OCD treatment

Down

1. Fear of being alone
3. Repetitive rituals to counteract anxiety
5. For example, "It's the OCD, not me"

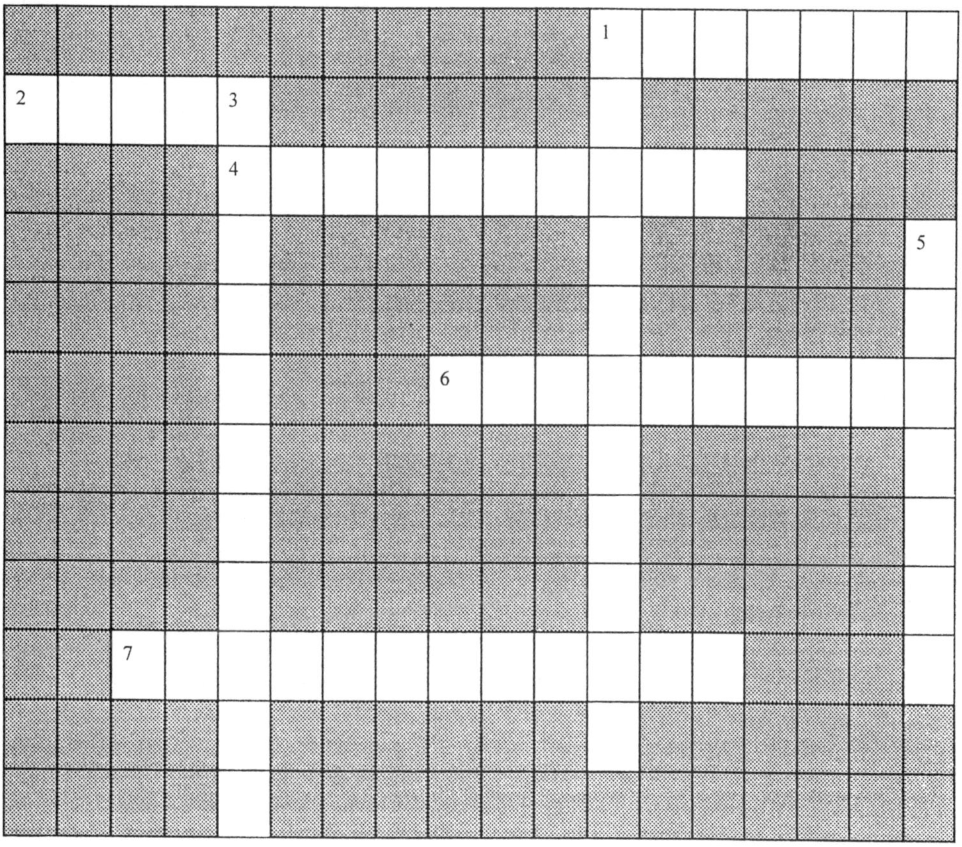

Fill in the blanks

Read each statement carefully and place the correct answer in the space(s) provided.

1. ______________ is a characteristic symptom of dissociative disorders.
2. For each symptom listed, identify if the symptom is physical, affective, cognitive, or behavioral
   a. Impatience ______________________________
   b. Hypervigilance ______________________________
   c. Shortness of breath ______________________________
   d. Distractibility ______________________________
   e. Speech dysfluency ______________________________
   f. Hypotension ______________________________
   g. Impaired coordination ______________________________
3. Patients with sleep panic attacks often develop ______________________________.
4. ______________ are three times more likely to experience panic disorders than ______________.
5. Electrical stimulation of ____________ gives rise to increased fears and anxiety.
6. Serotonin agonists appear to have ____________ and ____________ properties.

7. Severe stressors result in increased ____________ concentration in the hippocampus, amygdala, and locus ceruleus.
8. For each of the following concepts, identify the correct psychological theory of causation.
   a. Neurophysiologic vulnerability with disturbed parent-child relationships ____________
   b. Unconscious repression of instinctual sexual drives ____________
   c. Interoceptive conditioning ____________
9. Because of the need for higher doses of antidepressant medications to treat patients with panic disorder, the patient may have difficulty tolerating ____________ side effects.
10. The treatment of choice for agoraphobia is ____________.
11. With GAD, kindling results from ____________ of nerve cells via environmental stressors.
12. An abnormal sensitivity to ____________ has been evidenced in patients with GAD.
13. The most common obsession is focused on the fear of ____________.
14. The most effective agents used to treat OCD are ____________.
15. The essential feature of all dissociative disorders involves a failure to integrate ____________, ____________, and ____________.

Multiple choice

Circle the option that best answers the question.

1. For the patient receiving benzodiazepine for panic disorders, which of the following is the priority?
   a. Nutrition
   b. Rest
   c. Safety
   d. Activity
2. When dealing with a patient experiencing a panic attack, the nurse should do which of the following?
   a. Reassure the patient that the episode is not as bad as he thinks it is
   b. Place the patient in the day room with other patients watching television
   c. Explain what's happening in detail so the patient better understands
   d. Stay with him, recognizing his need to maintain personal space
3. A nurse is teaching a patient about the "4 square" method of breathing. Which of the following statements by the patient indicates effective instruction?
   a. "I'll inhale through my mouth and breath out through my nose."
   b. "I'll practice this technique whenever I'm anxious."
   c. "I'll do one controlled breath followed by 2 normal breaths."
   d. "I'll hold my breath to a count of 4 after exhaling."
4. When administering a TCA agent to a patient with a panic disorder, the nurse administers the drug once a day at bedtime based on the knowledge that sedating side effects will be lessened because of which of the following?
   a. Long half-life
   b. Enhanced absorption
   c. Prolonged metabolism
   d. Increased excretion
5. When administering combination therapy of antidepressants and high potency benzodiazepines, the nurse understands that this treatment protocol helps to:
   a. Minimize the complications of long-term antidepressant use
   b. Provide rapid symptom relief
   c. Reduce risk of withdrawal symptoms of both agents
   d. Decrease need for dietary restrictions
6. When interpreting the results of a patient's self-reporting rating scale, it is important for the nurse to remember which of the following?
   a. The patient's responses accurately represents his thoughts and feelings
   b. The patient is cognizant of his symptoms during an attack
   c. The patient's responses are usually similar to those of another patient
   d. The patient's awareness about feelings and events can be heightened
7. Based on the nurse's knowledge of alprazolam, the nurse would expect to administer the drug:
   a. Once daily in the morning
   b. Evenly divided doses throughout the day
   c. With breakfast and lunch
   d. Daily at bedtime

8. In an attempt to control his panic, a patient counters his negative thoughts of "I'm going to die" with "This is only anxiety and it will pass." The patient is using which of the following?
   a. Positive self-talk
   b. Distraction
   c. Systematic desensitization
   d. Implosive therapy
9. A patient diagnosed with GAD is placed on buspirone. The nurse instructs the patient that the drug's anxiolytic effects would be noticeable in approximately:
   a. 24 hours
   b. 1 week
   c. 2 weeks
   d. 1 month
10. When instructing a patient with GAD about nutrition therapy, the nurse is correct in advising the patient to avoid foods that contain which of the following?
    a. Tartrazine
    b. Tyramine
    c. Caffeine
    d. Sodium
11. When developing a teaching plan about the biochemical basis for OCD, an instructor includes a discussion about which of the following?
    a. GABA
    b. Serotonin
    c. Norepinephrine
    d. Cholecystokinin
12. In preparation for a class examination on anxiety disorders, a student is reviewing the theories of causation for OCD. The student is correct in identifying which of the following as associated with the behavioral theory?
    a. The more successful the compulsions are at relieving anxiety, the more they will continue
    b. A defense mechanism involving regression from oedipal to anal phase
    c. Carbon dioxide hypersensitivity resulting in hyperventilation
    d. Stages of anticipatory anxiety and phobic avoidance
13. When assessing a patient with OCD, the nurse anticipates a possible problem in which of the following areas?
    a. Nutrition
    b. Hygiene
    c. Cognition
    d. Elimination
14. A patient is hospitalized for treatment of OCD. Initially, the nurse should do which of the following?
    a. Restrict the patient for engaging in rituals
    b. Explain routines clearly and carefully
    c. Initiate behavioral treatment interventions
    d. Educate the patient about the basis for obsessions

Critical thinking exercises

1. Obtain a copy of the movie, *Copy Cat,* with Sigourney Weaver, available on videotape.
   a. After watching the movie, analyze the character played by Sigourney Weaver for key characteristics of panic disorder with agoraphobia.

   b. Evaluate her character for possible biopsychosocial etiologies for her disorder.

2. The following nursing diagnoses are identified on the plan of care for a patient with panic disorder. Identify defining characteristics for each nursing diagnosis and propose appropriate outcomes.

Nursing diagnosis	*Defining characteristics*	*Possible outcomes*
Anxiety		
Risk for self-harm		
Social isolation		
Powerlessness		
Disabling ineffective family coping		

3. Using the critical thinking dilemma in text box 17-6 (in the textbook), Joan with OCD, develop an appropriate plan of care that addresses the patient's needs and the staff's complaints.

4. As part of a class discussion, have a close friend or fellow classmate use the progressive muscle relaxation exercise found in text box 17-4 (in the textbook) on yourself. After the exercise, describe your thoughts, feelings, and perceptions, before, during, and after the exercise.

18 ▪ *Personality and impulse-control disorders*

CHAPTER HIGHLIGHTS

Chapter 18 explores the three clusters of personality disorders, (A, B, and C) and impulse-control disorders, including their common features and diagnostic criteria. It focuses primarily on Cluster B personality disorders, specifically, borderline and antisocial personality disorders. The chapter also addresses epidemiology, etiology, and nursing management of Cluster A and C disorders and reviews impulse-control disorders, such as intermittent explosive disorder, kleptomania, pyromania, pathologic gambling, and trichotillomania. Applying the nursing process with integration of the biopsychosocial framework, the chapter describes the nursing management of the patient with borderline and antisocial personality disorders.

Chapter 18 key points include the following:

- Personality, a complex pattern of characteristics, largely outside the person's awareness, comprise the individual's distinctive patterns of perceiving, feeling, thinking, coping, and behavior. It emerges from a complex interaction of biologic dispositions, psychological experiences, and environmental situations.
- Personality disorder is an enduring pattern of inner experiences and behavior, deviating markedly from the individual's cultural expectations. It is pervasive and inflexible with an onset in adolescence or early adulthood, stable over time, and leads to distress or impairment.
- Severity of personality disorders can be determined by tenuous stability, adaptive inflexibility, and vicious circles of rigid and inflexible behavior, resulting in serious interpersonal problems and social dysfunction.
- DSM IV classifies personality disorders on Axis II, organized around three clusters: A (odd-eccentric); B (dramatic-emotional); and C (anxious-fearful), any of which can coexist with Axis I disorders.
- Persons with borderline personality disorder have difficulty regulating emotion and have extreme fears of abandonment, leading to dysfunctional relationships and often engaging in self-injury.
- Antisocial personality disorders, often synonymous with psychopathology, includes individuals with no regard for and refusing to conform to social rules.
- Difficulties with emotional regulation or being able to recognize and control expression of feelings is seen with personality disorders. Education about communication skills and techniques, thought stopping techniques, distraction, or problem solving are effective in helping patients to identify feelings and gain control over them and their actions.
- Odd eccentric behaviors, seen with Cluster A personality disorders, often result in alienating the person from others. Social skills training, environmental management, and cognitive skill building may be helpful, with evaluation in terms of small changes in thinking and behavior.
- Cluster A disorders include paranoid (suspicious pattern), schizoid (asocial pattern), and schizotypal (eccentric) personality disorders.
- Cluster C personality, characterized by anxieties and fears include avoidant, dependent, and obsessive compulsive disorders. Obsessive compulsive personality disorder differs from OCD because the individual demonstrates an overall rigidity, perfectionism, and need for control.
- A therapeutic nurse-patient relationship, one of the most helpful interventions, provides the patient with a model of healthy interaction of trust, consistency, caring boundaries, and limita-

tions and helps the patient to build self-esteem and respect for self and others. A patient's avoidance of interpersonal and emotional attachment may interfere with developing a true therapeutic relationship.

- Inpatient treatment usually is necessary when patients experience periods of destructive behavior or self-harm. Treatment is usually delivered in the community over time. Continuity of care is important to help the individual change lifelong personality patterns.
- Impulse control disorders, not classified as personality disorders, share the same primary characteristic of impulsivity, leading to inappropriate social behaviors considered harmful to one's self and others, giving the patient the excitement or gratification at the time the act is committed.

STUDENT ACTIVITIES

Matching

Place the letter of the description from the righthand column next to the correct term in the lefthand column.

_______ 1. Dissociation
_______ 2. Emotions
_______ 3. Projective identification
_______ 4. Mindfulness
_______ 5. Tenuous stability
_______ 6. Trichotillomania
_______ 7. Temperament
_______ 8. Affective instability
_______ 9. Impulsivity
_______ 10. Dichotomous thinking
_______ 11. Pyromania
_______ 12. Adaptive inflexibility

a. Acting without considering the consequences of the action
b. Fragile personality pattern lacking resiliency under subjective stress
c. Rapid and extreme mood shifts
d. Rigidity in interactions with others, goal achievement and coping
e. Viewing things as absolute
f. Psychophysiologic reactions defining a person's mood
g Recognizable and distinctive way of behavior evidenced early in life
h. Irresistible impulse to start fires
i. Chronic self-destructive hair pulling
j. Psychological and behavioral version of meditation skills
k. Splitting of closely connected behaviors, thoughts, or feelings
l. Attributing own unacceptable feelings and impulses to another

Short answer

Write your answer to the question in the space provided.

1. Identify the ultimate treatment goal for a person diagnosed with histrionic personality disorder.

2. State the belief thought to be the basis of narcissistic personality disorder.

3. Name the most prominent feature of paranoid personality disorder.

4. Identify the primary focus of treatment for a person with schizoid personality disorder.

5. List the types of interventions from which a schizotypal personality disorder can benefit.

6. State the area in which patients with avoidant personality disorder exhibit sensitivity.

7. Identify the most frequent disorder encountered by therapists in their offices.

8. Name the two neurotransmitters associated with arson.

9. Describe the feeling that the person with trichotillomania experiences before and after the behavior.

10. List the four phases of pathologic gambling.

Multiple choice

Circle the option that best answers the question.

1. When reviewing a patient's chart, the nurse observes that the patient is diagnosed with paranoid personality disorder. The nurse is correct in identifying this as which of the following?
   a. Cluster A
   b. Cluster B
   c. Cluster C
   d. Factitious disorder
2. When dealing with a patient with a personality disorder, it is important that the nurse remembers that:
   a. The change in the patient's behavior typically occurs quickly
   b. The patient is able to control the pattern of behavior
   c. The patient's behavior often provokes negative feelings in others
   d. Once alerted to the behavior problem, the patient can change the behavior
3. While assessing a patient with a suspected personality disorder, the nurse would expect to find which of the following?
   a. Flexibility in coping
   b. Socially appropriate reactions
   c. Ability to learn new coping skills
   d. Self-defeating circle of events
4. During an interview, a patient states, "I became a lawyer because my father wanted me to be one." The nurse interprets this statement as indicative of which of the following?
   a. Affective instability
   b. Identity diffusion
   c. Dissociation
   d. Tenuous stability
5. A patient diagnosed with borderline personality disorder states, "I'm so ugly, who'd want to go out with me. I can't even do my job. Why wouldn't I get reprimanded by my boss." The nurse correctly interprets this as a maladaptive schema in which of the following domains?
   a. Autonomy
   b. Connectedness
   c. Worthiness
   d. Expectations and limits
6. Which of the following questions by the nurse would help elicit information about dichotomous thinking?
   a. "What do you think about those with whom you work?"
   b. "Have you ever been hurt by your spur of the moment action?"
   c. "Was there ever a time you didn't remember events around you?"
   d. "What makes you feel happy, sad?"
7. When planning care for a patient with borderline personality disorder, which of the following nursing diagnoses is a priority?
   a. Altered thought processes
   b. Personal identity disturbance
   c. Sleep pattern disturbance
   d. Risk for self-mutilation
8. A patient with borderline personality disorder and transient psychotic episodes involving voices is being discharged home. Which of the following instructions by the nurse is appropriate for helping the patient deal with these episodes?
   a. Take an additional dose of your medication to control the voices
   b. Tell yourself, " I'm not hearing voices"
   c. Call the clinic immediately and ask to speak to the nurse on call
   d. Watch some television to distract yourself

9. When establishing a therapeutic nurse-patient relationship with a patient with borderline personality disorder, it is important for the nurse to do which of the following?
   a. Tell the patient that the relationship will last as long as necessary
   b. Respect the patient's boundaries at all times
   c. Limit interactions to 30 minutes or less
   d. Aggressively confront the patient about boundary violations
10. When dealing with a patient with an antisocial personality disorder, the nurse understands that the patient's need for independence is based on which of the following?
   a. Belief in own self-worth
   b. Rewards for competitive behavior
   c. Inability to delay gratification
   d. Sense of mistrust of others
11. When teaching a patient with antisocial personality disorder, the nurse should:
   a. Be direct and firm with the patient
   b. Lecture the patient about the behavior
   c. Bargain with the patient about rules
   d. Allow the patient to direct discussions
12. When caring for the patient with schizoid personality disorder, the nurse primarily focuses on which of the following?
   a. Increasing solitary activities
   b. Increasing patient's ability to feel pleasure
   c. Maintaining patient's emotional responsiveness to others
   d. Expanding the patient's interest in objects and things
13. When interacting with a patient diagnosed with dependent personality disorder, the nurse should do which of the following?
   a. Tell the patient what to do
   b. Teach appropriate functional skills
   c. Make any decisions for the patient
   d. Anticipate need for antidepressant therapy

Critical thinking exercises

1. A patient diagnosed with borderline personality disorder has the following nursing diagnoses identified on the plan of care. Identify possible defining characteristics and propose appropriate outcomes for each.

Nursing diagnosis	*Defining characteristics*	*Possible outcomes*
Anxiety		
Dysfunctional grieving		
Risk for loneliness		
Personal identity disturbance		

2. Analyze the clinical vignette, Joanne Smith, found in text box 18-3 (in the textbook), and develop an appropriate plan of care that addresses this patient's priority needs.

3. Using the patient scenario presented in Nursing Care Plan 18-1 (in the textbook), Yolanda Jones, and the chart below, synthesize possible biopsychosocial etiologies for this patient from your analysis and develop appropriate biopsychosocial outcomes and interventions.

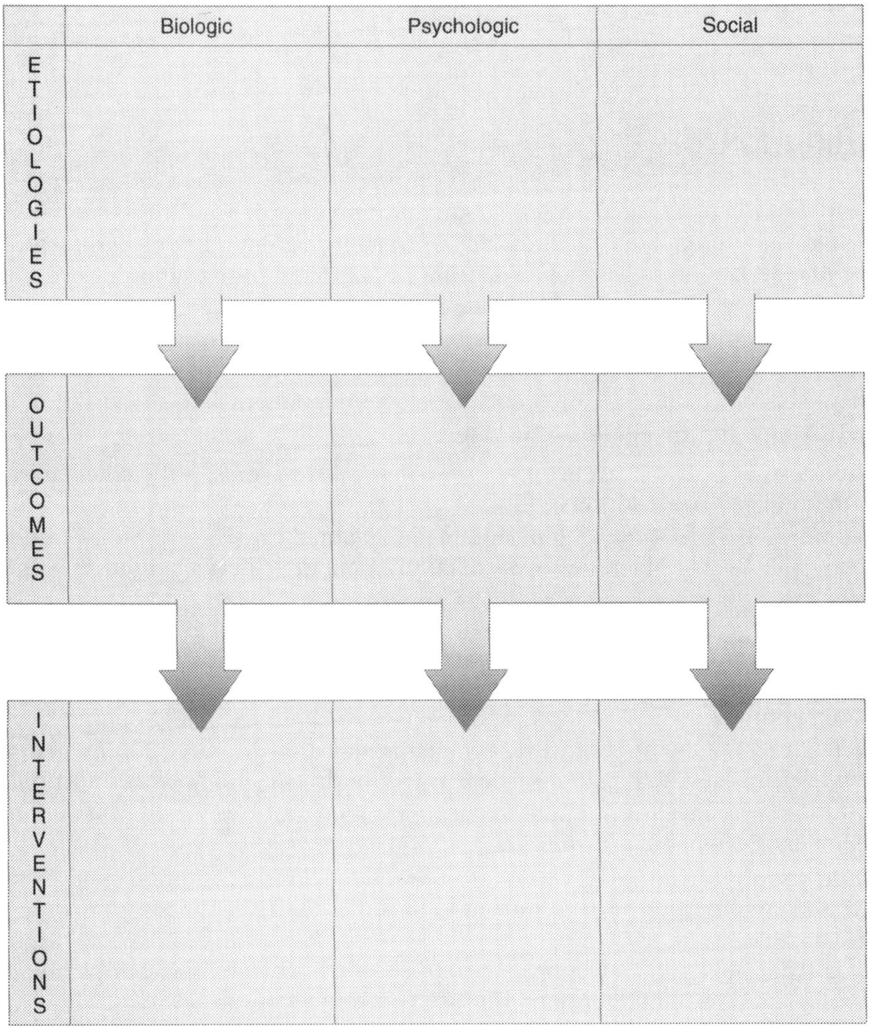

4. As part of an assignment, you are asked to lead a class discussion comparing and contrasting the key characteristics and associated findings of obsessive compulsive personality disorder and OCD. Create a chart that you can distribute to your fellow classmates for the discussion.

19 ▪ *Somatoform and related disorders*

CHAPTER HIGHLIGHTS

Chapter 19 explores the psychiatric diagnosis, somatization disorder and reviews other somatoform disorders such as undifferentiated somatoform, conversion, pain, and body dysmorphic disorders, hypochondriasis, and factitious disorders. Focusing primarily on somatization disorder this chapter examines the epidemiology, including distribution, age of onset, gender, ethnic, and cultural differences, and comorbidity, and addresses possible etiologic theories of causation, risk factors, and somatic interventions. Applying the nursing process with integration of the biopsychosocial framework, this chapter describes the nursing management of the patient with somatization disorder.

Chapter 19 key points include the following:

- Somatization, psychological stress manifested in physical symptoms, is the chief characteristics of somatoform and factitious disorders.
- With somatoform disorders, the patient suffers unexplained physical symptoms but does not self inflict injury, whereas with factitious disorders, the patient self-inflicts injuries to gain medical attention.
- Sociocultural and gender factors have been associated with somatization disorder, occurring more frequently in women, those less educated, those living in urban areas, and those who are older, separated, widowed, or divorced. It is more common in Mexican-American women than non-Hispanic women.
- There are 6 clusters of clinical syndromes: somatization disorder; undifferentiated somatoform disorder; conversion disorder; pain disorder; hypochondriasis; and body dysmorphic disorder.
- Somatization disorder involves multiple physical problems and symptoms; other clinical subtypes involve recurrence of one major symptom.
- Somatization disorders, the most complex, is a chronic, relapsing condition characterized by multiple physical symptoms that develop during times of emotional distress, occurring primarily in women.
- Factitious disorders include two types: factitious disorder in which physical or psychological symptoms (or both) are fabricated to assume the sick role and factitious disorder NOS.
- Many complexities in identifying and diagnosing patients with somatoform and factitious disorders exist because the patients refuse to accept any psychiatric basis for their problems. They often go years moving from one health care provider to another to receive medical attention and avoid psychiatric assessment. Finally, they receive mental health treatment because of comorbid conditions, such as depression or panic.
- Development of the nurse-patient relationship is crucial. Nurses need a flexible relaxed nonjudgmental approach that acknowledges the symptoms but focuses on new ways of coping with stress and avoiding recurrence of symptoms.
- Health teaching is important in helping the individual develop positive lifestyle changes. Identification of personal strengths and supporting positive skill development improves self-esteem and personal confidence. Education about biofeedback and relaxation provides the patient with positive coping skills.

STUDENT ACTIVITIES

Word unscramble

Below is a list of scrambled words. Unscramble each word and place it in the appropriate space next to its definition.

isaishpochryond   tioninretnzalia

itcmaosohcyps   alnerimigng

noitzatamosi

______________ 1. Preoccupation with fears about developing a serious illness based on one's misinterpretation of body sensations.

______________ 2. Manifestation of physical symptoms resulting from psychological distress.

______________ 3. Process of coping with life problems or stressors by expressing anxiety, stress, and frustration through own physical symptoms.

______________ 4. Conditions in which a psychological state contributes to the development of a physical illness.

______________ 5. Intentional production of illness symptoms motivated by a specific self-serving goal.

Labeling

On the biopsychosocial etiology figure below, write the letter of the corresponding statement about the causative theory in the appropriate circle.

a. Familial tendency
b. Choice of spouse with antisocial personality disorder
c. Substitution for repressed impulses
d. Form of social or emotional communication
e. View of mind-body distinction in the Western world
f. Left hemispheric dysfunction

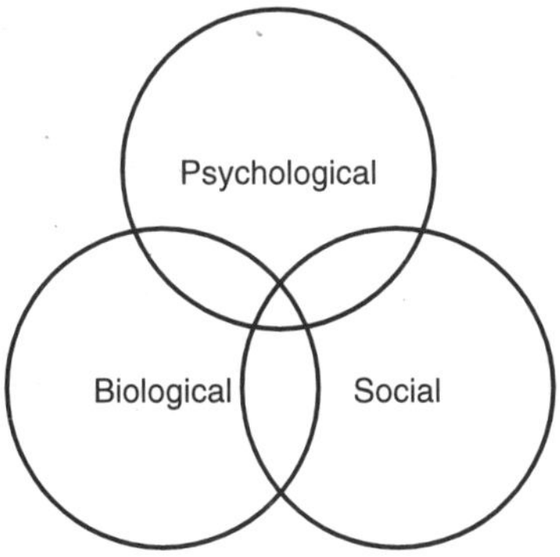

Multiple choice

Circle the option that best answers the question.

1. A patient diagnosed with somatization disorder is being treated with phenelzine for depression experiences a hypertensive crisis. The nurse would anticipate administering:
   a. Nifedipine
   b. Phentolamine
   c. Busiprone
   d. Diazepam

2. When assessing a patient with suspected somatization disorder, the nurse would expect to find which of the following?
   a. Unconcern about the physical symptoms
   b. Report of fluctuating and changing symptoms
   c. Statements of overall poor health
   d. High functional ability

3. When performing the psychological assessment of a patient with somatization disorder, the nurse would expect to find?
   a. Flat affect
   b. Impaired cognition
   c. Delusional thinking
   d. Labile mood
4. When communicating with a patient with somatization disorder, the nurse should focus the interaction on:
   a. Pharmacologic therapy
   b. Physical symptoms
   c. Psychosocial problems
   d. Daily routines
5. A patient in the ambulatory care setting complains of urinary retention, visual problems, difficulty swallowing, and coordination problems. No physiologic cause can be determined. Based on the findings, the nurse would anticipate the possibility of which of the following?
   a. Conversion disorder
   b. Undifferentiated somatoform disorder
   c. Pain disorder
   d. Hypochondriasis
6. Which of the following statements would alert the nurse to the possibility of body dysmorphic disorder?
   a. " I know I have pneumonia. This cough is terrible."
   b. "My hands are so disfigured. I wear gloves all the time."
   c. "I'm always just so tired, I don't know why."
   d. "How can I function with this headache?"
7. When teaching a group of students about how factitious disorders differ from somatoform disorders, the instructor is correct in explaining that which of the following is true about factitious disorders?
   a. The cause of the illness is unintentional
   b. Motivation focuses on dependency of health care providers
   c. Unexplainable psychological symptoms predominate
   d. Symptoms are localized to one body system
8. A patient is brought to the hospital by her mother. History reveals numerous previous hospitalizations for the child, requiring diagnostic tests and surgical procedures for a variety of problems. The mother has been caring for the patient, such as administering injections for antibiotic therapy and performing intermittent catheterization for voiding problems. After careful review of the patient's record, it is determined that the mother is inflicting the problems on the child. The nurse correctly identifies this as which of the following?
   a. Munchausen by proxy
   b. Conversion disorder
   c. Body dysmorphic disorder
   d. Malingering

Critical thinking exercises

1. Use the clinical vignette found in text box 19-1 (in the textbook), Mrs. A.
   a. Develop a therapeutic dialogue with this patient that would be effective in eliciting important information.

   b. Develop an appropriate plan of care based on an analysis of this patient's needs.

2. A 12-year-old female was involved in a school bus accident. No one was seriously hurt. The children experienced minor bumps and bruises, including the girl who bumped her knees on the seat back in front of her. After being at school all day, the girl stayed after school to watch a field hockey game and was driven home by her friend's parents. The next morning, while getting dressed for school, the girl complained of abdominal pain, nausea, and dizziness. She described the pain as sharp at times, coming and going, increasing after eating. She was initially seen by her family doctor, who could find no physiological basis for her complaints.

   The complaints continued for two months, during which time the girl remained at home. The parents were concerned because at the age of 10, this child had undergone an exploratory laparotomy with removal of both ovaries and fallopian tubes because of a malignant ovarian tumor. Afterwards the parents doted on the child, with the parents attentively indulging the child when she complained of any illness.

   The child was taken to a variety of specialists and underwent numerous tests, all of which were within normal limits.

a. Based on your analysis of this situation, explain what is occurring.

b. Analyze the above situation for possible biopsychosocial etiologies and develop appropriate biopsychosocial outcomes and interventions for this patient.

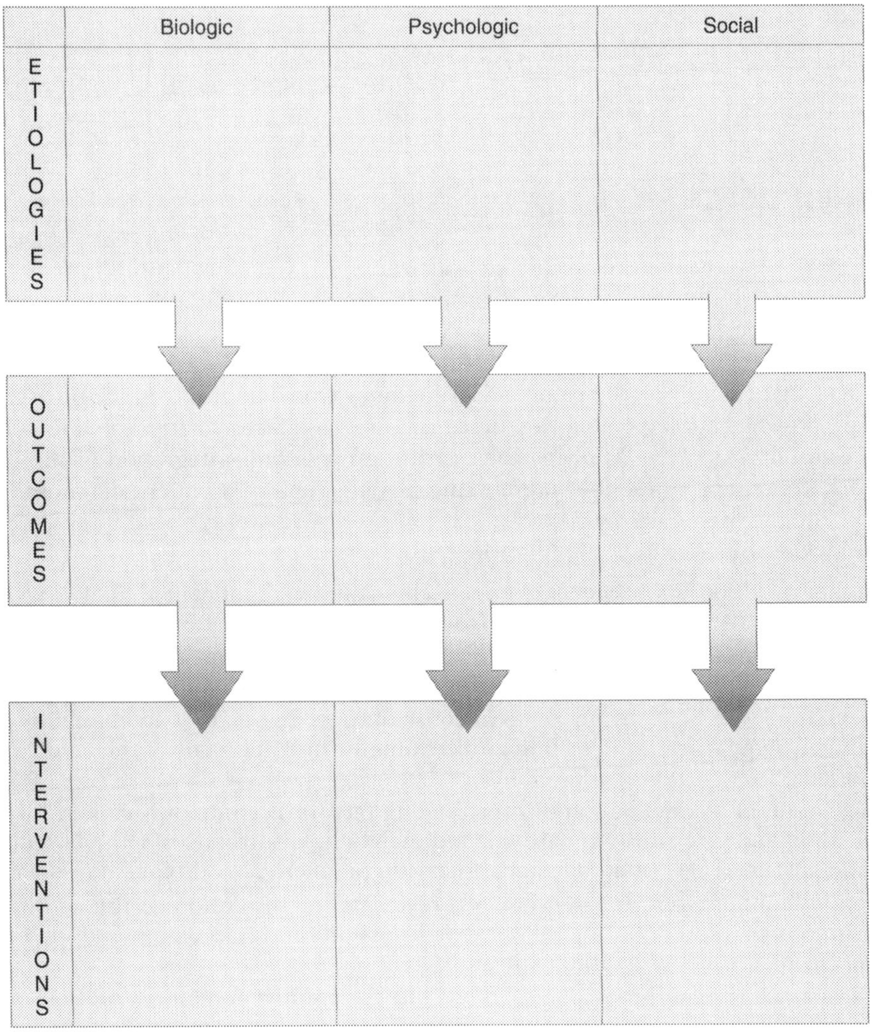

3. Imagine if you were assigned to care for the following patient. A 20-year-old female comes to the health clinic for a routine checkup. During the physical examination, the patient states, " Look at my breasts. They're so small. None of my clothes fit properly. I'm ashamed to wear a bathing suit out in public. In fact, I won't even go to my health club to work out because I'm so embarrassed about how I look." On observation, you note that although small, the patient's breasts are appropriate for the patient's body size and weight.

   a. Based on your knowledge of somatoform and factitious disorders, evaluate this patient's complaints.

   b. Develop a therapeutic dialogue that addresses this patient's needs.

20 ▪ *Neuropsychiatric disorders*

CHAPTER HIGHLIGHTS

Chapter 20 explores the neuropsychiatric disorders of delirium and dementia, primarily Alzheimer's type dementia. It also reviews other dementias including vascular dementia, those caused by other medical conditions, such as HIV, head trauma, Parkinson's disease, Huntington's disease, Pick's disease, and Creutzfeldt-Jakob disease, substance-induced dementia, and amnesiac disorders. Focusing primarily on delirium and Alzheimer's type dementia, this chapter examines the epidemiology, possible etiologic theories of causation, risk factors, and somatic interventions, including psychopharmacology. Applying the nursing process with integration of the biopsychosocial framework, this chapter describes the nursing management of a patient diagnosed with either delirium or Alzheimer's type dementia.

Chapter 20 key points include the following:

- Neuropsychiatric disorders are characterized clinically by significant deficits in cognition or memory that represent a clear-cut change from a previous level of functioning.
- Two major syndromes, delirium and chronic cognitive impairments, such as dementia, occur in the elderly. Interventions and outcomes differ for each syndrome.
- Delirium, characterized by a disturbance in consciousness and change in cognition over a short period of time, requires rapid detection and treatment. In 25 percent of the cases, it is a sign of impending death.
- Delirium, a result of a combination of precipitating factors, is commonly caused by medication, infections, fluid and electrolyte imbalance, and metabolic disturbances. Other predisposing factors include advanced age, brain damage, preexisting dementia, and biopsychosocial stressors.
- The primary treatment goal for delirium is prevention or resolution of the acute confusional episode with return to previous cognitive status. Interventions focus on elimination or correction of the underlying cause and symptomatic and safety supportive measures.
- Dementia, characterized by gradual onset of decline in cognitive function, especially memory and usually accompanied by changes in personality and behavior, has numerous causes. Some are irreversible, such as hypoxia, carbon monoxide poisoning, and vitamin deficiencies.
- Alzheimer's disease is an example of a progressive, degenerative dementia. Treatment currently focuses on reducing cognitive symptoms in an attempt to improve the quality of life for the patient and caregivers.
- No one cause for dementia and Alzheimer's disease has been discovered. Research, which continues to pinpoint a single identifiable genetic basis, is also focusing on other implicated etiologies such as neurochemical, neuropathologic, and some environmental factors.
- Some psychosocial stressors are known to precipitate delirium or contribute to worsening dementia. These include sensory over- or underload, immobilization, sleep deprivation, fatigue, pain or hunger, changes in routine, or demands beyond the patient's ability. Nursing intervention focuses on reducing the impact of these stressors and educating caregivers and families.
- Education about what to expect, progressive cognitive decline and behavior changes, environmental safety, and community resources is essential.
- Symptoms of dementia may also result from a number of disorders, such as vascular and amnesiac disorders, head trauma, HIV, and substance abuse. Dementia may also appear as a symptoms of Parkinson's, Huntington's, Pick's, and Creutzfeldt-Jakob diseases.

STUDENT ACTIVITIES

Word find

Hidden within the following letter grid are key terms from chapter 20, listed below. The terms may be vertical, horizontal, diagonal, or backward. Circle the words as you find them.

Agnosia	Delirium
Aphasia	Dementia
Apraxia	Memory
Bradykinesia	Neuropsychiatry
Cognition	Pick's disease

T	A	M	U	I	R	I	L	E	D
A	I	S	O	N	G	A	B	A	A
E	T	M	M	E	M	P	O	I	I
S	N	I	X	U	D	R	S	A	S
A	E	N	A	R	Y	A	R	R	E
E	M	E	I	O	H	X	O	Y	N
S	E	U	P	P	A	I	P	O	I
I	D	R	A	S	S	A	T	R	K
D	U	O	C	Y	H	Y	A	H	Y
S	O	I	O	C	K	I	C	K	D
K	P	G	R	H	S	A	H	I	A
C	O	G	N	I	T	I	O	N	R
I	O	I	N	A	L	F	F	E	B
P	K	G	I	T	K	E	I	S	R
T	A	T	N	R	O	S	D	Y	A
D	E	M	E	Y	R	O	M	E	M

Matching

Place the letter of the description from the righthand columnn next to the correct term in the left-hand column.

_______ 1. Cognition
_______ 2.. Cortical dementia
_______ 3. Korsakoff syndrome
_______ 4. Progressive illness
_______ 5. Delirium
_______ 6. Memory
_______ 7. Multi-infarct dementia
_______ 8. Subcortical dementia

a. Vascular dementia with resulting brain damage form TIAs
b. Disturbance in consciousness and changes in cognition developing over a short period of time
c. Dysfunction or deterioration of the brain's deep gray or white matter structures.
d. Dysfunction characterizes by amnesia, aphasia, apraxia, and agnosia
e. Profound deficit in ability to form new memories with some associated deficit in recall of old memories despite a clear sensorium
f. Disorder continually advancing or worsening
g. High level of intellectual processing involving acquisition, use, or manipulation of perceptions and information
h. Ability to recall or reproduce learning and experiences

Multiple choice

Circle the option that best answers the question.

1. When assessing a patient's risk for delirium, the nurse would be especially alert for an increased risk in which of the following patients?
   a. Elderly postoperative male patient with severe pain
   b. Female patient newly diagnosed with AIDs
   c. A middle-aged female with a fractured hip
   d. A young adult male dehydrated from gastroenteritis
2. A patient diagnosed with delirium is to receive medication therapy. The nurse anticipates that the physician most probably will order which of the following?
   a. Lorazepam
   b. Fluoxetine
   c. Haloperidol
   d. Chlorpromazine
3. An instructor is explaining the differences between delirium and dementia to a group of students. When explaining about delirium, the instructor is correct in stating which of the following?
   a. The onset is slow and changes from day to day
   b. Immediate and recent memory is usually severely impaired
   c. The patient is disoriented to person, place, and time
   d. Tremors and hyperactivity are often absent
4. When caring for the patient with delirium, which of the following interventions takes priority?
   a. Discontinuing all medications
   b. Applying restraints
   c. Providing for adequate nutrition
   d. Interacting frequently with reorientation
5. During a family support group meeting, one of the members asks the leader, "What causes Alzheimer's disease?" The leader is correct in replying:
   a. "The disorder is passed on by genes."
   b. "An enzyme for a neurochemical is decreased."
   c. "A virus in the environment causes degeneration."
   d. "The exact cause is not known right now."
6. The physician orders donepozil (Aricept), 5 mg, for a patient diagnosed with Alzheimer's type dementia. When administering the drug, the nurse understands that this drug acts to:
   a. Reduce the amount of calcium entering the cell
   b. Inhibit cholinesterase in the central nervous system
   c. Mimic the action of acetylcholine
   d. Slow the breakdown of acetylcholine
7. The daughter of a patient with Alzheimer's type dementia reports increasing agitation, anxiety, and restlessness, especially when she asks her mother to get washed and dressed. Suddenly one day, the patient wandered away from home. The nurse interprets this as which of the following?
   a. Catastrophic response
   b. Depression
   c. Delirium
   d. Psychosis
8. The nurse is developing an activity program for a patient with Alzheimer's disease. When instituting this plan, the nurse should do which of the following?
   a. Confront the patient about problems he is having
   b. Allow the patient to direct the activity
   c. Offer simple directions the patient can master
   d. Show the patient how to do it first, then have him do it
9. A patient with progressive dementia is hyperactive. Which of the following nutritional instructions would be appropriate for his caregiver?
   a. "Make sure to include foods that are low protein and high fat to provide him energy."
   b. "Have him carry some bananas or breakfast bars with him so he can snack throughout the day."
   c. "Stick to offering him thick liquids or semisoft foods, like mashed potatoes and ground meat."
   d. "Limit the amount of milk-based foods, like ice cream and yogurt, that he consumes."

10. On a recent home visit, the caregiver reported to the nurse that her mother diagnosed with dementia was experiencing urinary incontinence throughout the day. The nurse instructed the caregiver on various strategies to help with this. On the next visit, the nurse evaluates the caregiver's response to the instructions. Which of the following statements would indicate to the nurse that the caregiver needs further instructions?
    a. "I've put a sign and picture on the bathroom door."
    b. "I've limited the amount of fluids she's been drinking."
    c. "I make sure that she wears easy to pull-on pants."
    d. "I put a commode next to her bed."
11. The physician orders tacrine (Cognex) for a patient with Alzheimer's type dementia. When administering this drug, the nurse should do which of the following?
    a. Administer the drug with meals
    b. Strop the drug immediately if a headache or fatigue develops
    c. Give the dosage as directed in the early morning
    d. Obtain baseline liver functions test before the first dose
12. A patient with dementia is scheduled for an invasive procedure. When preparing the patient, the nurse should do which of the following?
    a. Attempt to reason with the patient about the necessity of the treatment
    b. Orient the patient to the reality of the situation
    c. Explain the test in detail well in advance of the procedure
    d. Simply explain about the test immediately before it is to occur
13. When assessing a patient with multi-infarct dementia, the nurse understands that the greatest risk factor for this type of dementia is:
    a. Hypertension
    b. Diabetes
    c. Heart disease
    d. Chronic alcohol abuse

Critical thinking exercises

1. Attend an Alzheimer's support group and interview a caregiver(s) of a patient with Alzheimer's type dementia. Examine the issues and problems that the caregivers deal with every day and the methods they use to cope with these.

2. The nursing diagnoses identified on the plan of care for a patient with delirium are listed below. Identify possible defining characteristics and propose appropriate outcomes for each.

Nursing diagnosis	*Defining characteristics*	*Possible outcomes*
Acute confusion		
Sensory perceptual alterations		
Risk for violence (self-directed or directed at others)		
Impaired verbal communication		

3. Using the patient scenario presented in Nursing Care Plan 20-1 (in the textbook), Lois W., and the chart below, synthesize possible biopsychosocial etiologies for this patient from your analysis and develop appropriate biopsychosocial outcomes and interventions.

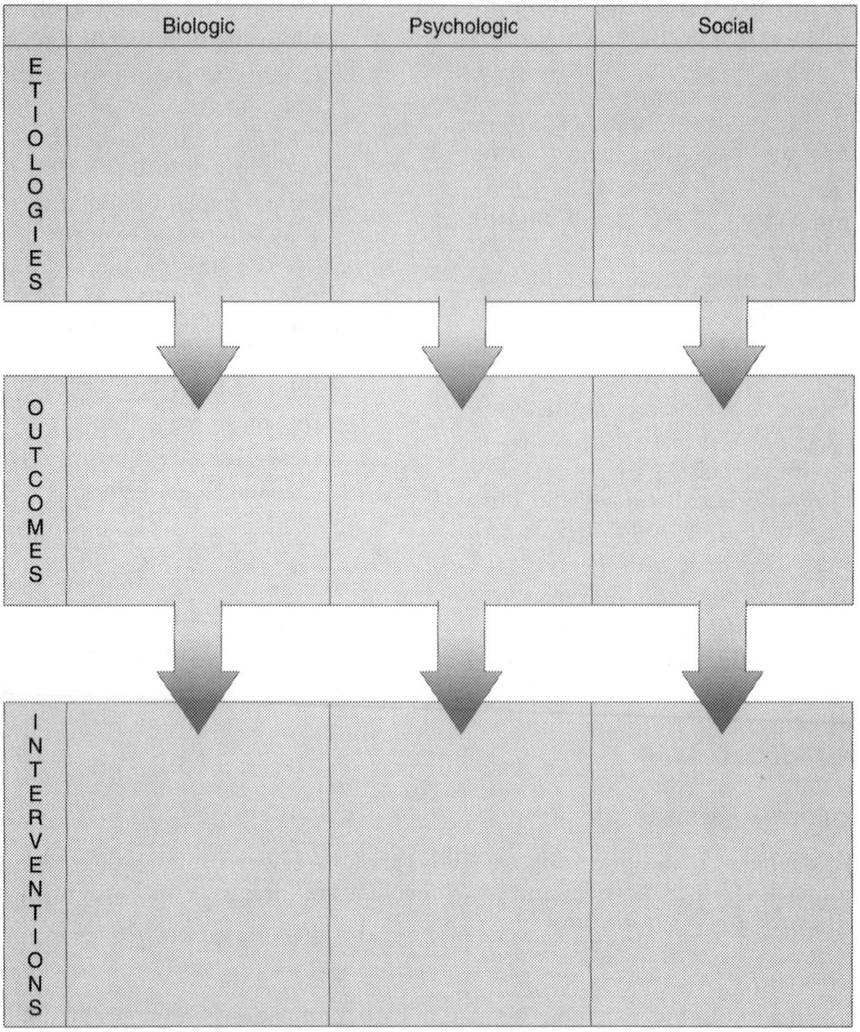

4. Visit a local long-term care facility and interview the nursing care coordinator. Investigate the number of patients currently admitted there that have a diagnosis of delirium or dementia.

   a. Analyze the measures used to maintain a safe, therapeutic environment.

   b. Develop a class presentation that addresses the measures used and also include suggestions for additional measures.

21 ▪ *Eating disorders*

CHAPTER HIGHLIGHTS

Chapter 21 explores the two major eating disorders—anorexia nervosa and bulimia nervosa. Using the biopsychosocial framework, the chapter reviews the major concepts, epidemiology, etiology, and psychopharmacologic interventions and applies the nursing process in the management of each disorder.

Chapter 21 key points include the following:

- Eating disorders primarily affect women in adolescence and young adulthood. Anorexia appears to peak in adolescence whereas bulimia appears to affect women in their early twenties.
- Patients with either disorder share similarities in psychological motivations, such as body image disturbance and gender identity problems.
- According to DSM IV criteria, anorexia is identified by the severity of weight loss (less than 85 percent of expected body weight for age and height) and accompanying amenorrhea. Bulimia is identified by the frequency of binge eating and inappropriate compensatory behaviors (at least twice a week over three months).
- Most patients experience both disorders simultaneously. Almost half of those with anorexia will develop symptoms of bulimia within two years.
- Patients with anorexia suggest more serious physiological disturbances associated with starvation often requiring hospitalization. Prognosis for recovery are less encouraging.
- A link between mood and biochemical changes on appetite and weight has been demonstrated. Substances such as norepinephrine, serotonin, dopamine, various neuropeptides, and some neuroendocrine hormones are thought to interact, thus influencing eating behavior.
- Disturbances of body image and gender identity, typical of individuals with eating disorders, are believed, in part, to be a result of the mixed societal and cultural messages about the female role and identity, emphasizing thinness and the perfect body.
- Similar patterns of family dynamics also have been found.
- Families of individuals with anorexia are characterized by enmeshment and a need to avoid conflict. Family members are rigid, methodical, obsessive, and hypersensitive to rejection or disapproval from others.
- Families of individuals with bulimia are more overly conflictual and demonstrate greater open hostility, criticism, and rejection of its members.
- Interventions for those with eating disorders focus on establishing a healing relationship between patient and nurse, establishing and maintaining regular adequate nutritional eating habits, interrupting the binge-purge cycle, restoring normal endocrine function, and teaching about normal physiologic weight regulation and adequate nutrition.

STUDENT ACTIVITIES

Fill in the blanks

Read each statement carefully and place the correct answer in the space(s) provided.

1. The process of ____________ entails fulfilling the set of culturally determined qualities and roles consistent with one being male or female.

2. ______________ refers to the mental picture of one's own body.
3. In studies with patients with anorexia, the rise in levels of ____________ in response to eating is lower during periods of starvation.
4. Increased levels of ___________ are linked positively to increased satiety.
5. The medication ______________ has been shown to be effective during the maintenance phase of treatment for anorexia.
6. The most common physical symptom of anorexia is ______________________________.
7. Because of lowered ____________ levels with malnutrition, use of antidepressants may produce more profound side effects.
8. Using the techniques of ______________ may help identify emotional triggers to disordered eating.
9. Bulimia is associated with a _____________ cycle.
10. The medication _____________ may be contraindicated for bulimic symptoms because of the higher incidence of grand mal seizures associated with its use.

Crossword puzzle

Across

3. Musculoskeletal symptom of weight loss
5. Lack of clear generational boundaries
6. Binge-purge cycle disorder
7. SSRI drug used for treatment
8. Dental enamel erosion

Down

1. Decreased platelet count
2. Levels rise in response to eating
4. Internal signal of having enough to eat
9. Fine, baby-like hair

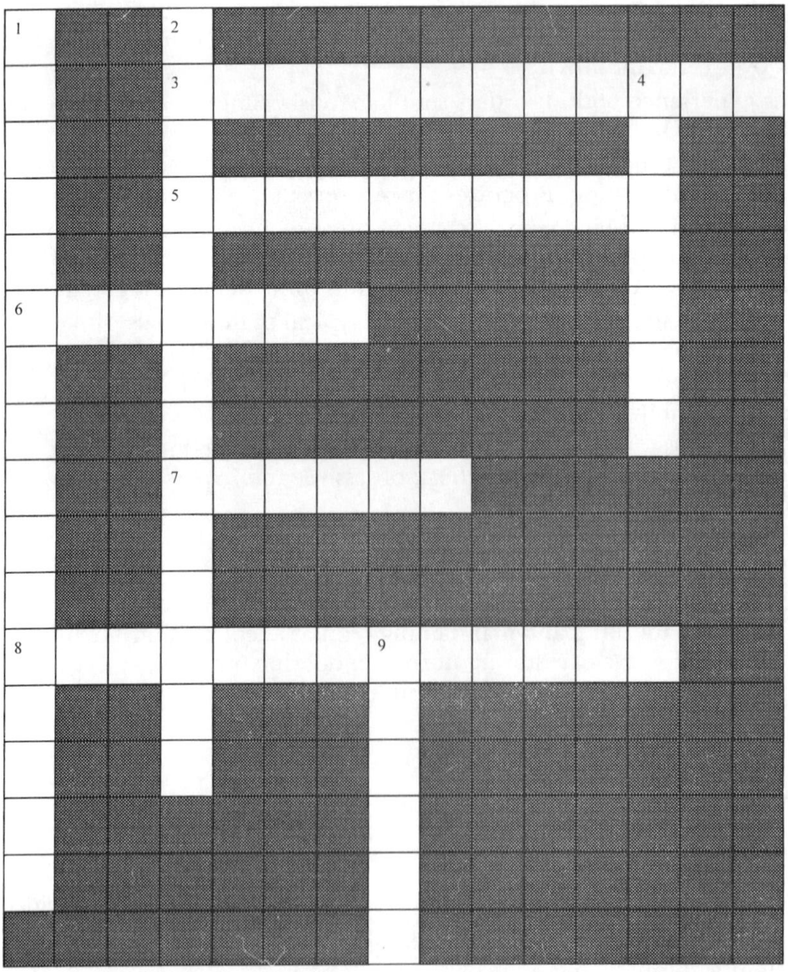

Multiple choice

Circle the option that best answers the question.

1. A patient with bulimia is receiving fluoxetine. The nurse explains to the patient and family that the full effect of the drug occurs:
   a. Immediately
   b. After approximately 1 week
   c. In approximately 4 weeks
   d. In approximately 4 months
2. A patient admitted to the hospital for dehydration and hypokalemia is suspected of having anorexia nervosa. The nurse understands that this diagnosis is based on which of the following criteria?
   a. Strong need to control the environment
   b. Body weight less than 85 percent of expected body weight for age and height
   c. Recurrent episodes of binge eating
   d. Inappropriate compensatory behaviors to prevent the gain of weight
3. For the patient with bulimia, the nurse is planning to include the family in therapy sessions. In doing so, the nurse remembers that families of individuals with bulimia tend to be:
   a. Enmeshed
   b. Overly sensitive
   c. Rigid and unchanging
   d. Perfect, overprotective
4. A patient with anorexia, known to purge by vomiting, is receiving antidepressant therapy. The nurse needs to assess this patient frequently for which of the following?
   a. Dyspepsia
   b. Constipation
   c. Orthostatic hypotension
   d. Flu-like symptoms
5. A patient being started on SSRI therapy complains of gastrointestinal symptoms associated with the drug. Which of the following instructions would be most helpful?
   a. "Eat small amounts of carbohydrates throughout the day."
   b. "Take the drug before you eat breakfast."
   c. "You need a stronger dosage. Let me call the doctor."
   d. "Try taking the drug at bedtime with a glass of milk."
6. Which of the following is a priority when caring for the patient with anorexia?
   a. Improving nutritional status
   b. Acknowledging the severity of the illness
   c. Identifying beliefs about body size
   d. Establishing a trusting relationship
7. The nurse is preparing a patient with bulimia for discharge. Which of the following statements by the patient indicates effective teaching?
   a. "I'll watch my intake of carbohydrates and fats."
   b. "I'll eat small meals and snacks regularly."
   c. "I know if I eat pasta, I'll binge."
   d. "I'll take my medication when I feel the urge to binge."
8. A patient with bulimia nervosa regularly engages in purging behaviors with self-induced vomiting. As a result of this behavior, which of the following laboratory test results might the nurse expect to see?
   a. Metabolic alkalosis
   b. Metabolic acidosis
   c. Low serum T3 levels
   d. Low serum estrogen levels
9. According to the learning theory, eating disorders are the result of which of the following?
   a. Confusion and conflicting feelings about one's own sexuality and gender identity
   b. Conflicting messages from society about roles and functions in life
   c. Inability to deal with increasing autonomy and psychosexual desires
   d. Conflict of independence of adolescence threatening affiliation and relationships
10. In addition to significant weight loss, which of the following symptoms might alert the nurse to suspect anorexia nervosa?
    a. Seizures
    b. Amenorrhea
    c. Constipation
    d. Bradycardia

Critical thinking exercises

1. Develop a chart identifying the biochemical changes associated with eating disorders and describe the role(s) each play in the development of an eating disorder.

2. Have a friend or family member take the eating attitudes test found in text box 21-4 (in the textbook). Score the test and draw a conclusion based on the person's score.

3. Imagine if a friend asks you to help out with teaching a health education class to a coed group of freshmen-level high school students. The topic is healthy nutrition. Develop a teaching plan that addresses this age group's needs and risks for possible eating disorders.

4. Pretend that you are a school nurse performing routine yearly health evaluations. You notice that a student has lost a significant amount of weight in the last six months. She appears thin and pale, wearing a turtleneck sweater, blouse, and loose cardigan sweater with loose, baggy jeans. When asked about her weight loss, she states, "I've been exercising a lot to lose weight because I'm so fat." After reviewing her records, you note that before her weight loss, her body weight was appropriate for her height. How would you approach this situation and how best can you intervene?

5. Using the patient scenario, Julie, the patient with anorexia nervosa, found in Nursing Care Plan 21-1 (in the textbook), and the chart below, identify possible biopsychosocial etiologies for this patient and develop appropriate biopsychosocial outcomes and interventions.

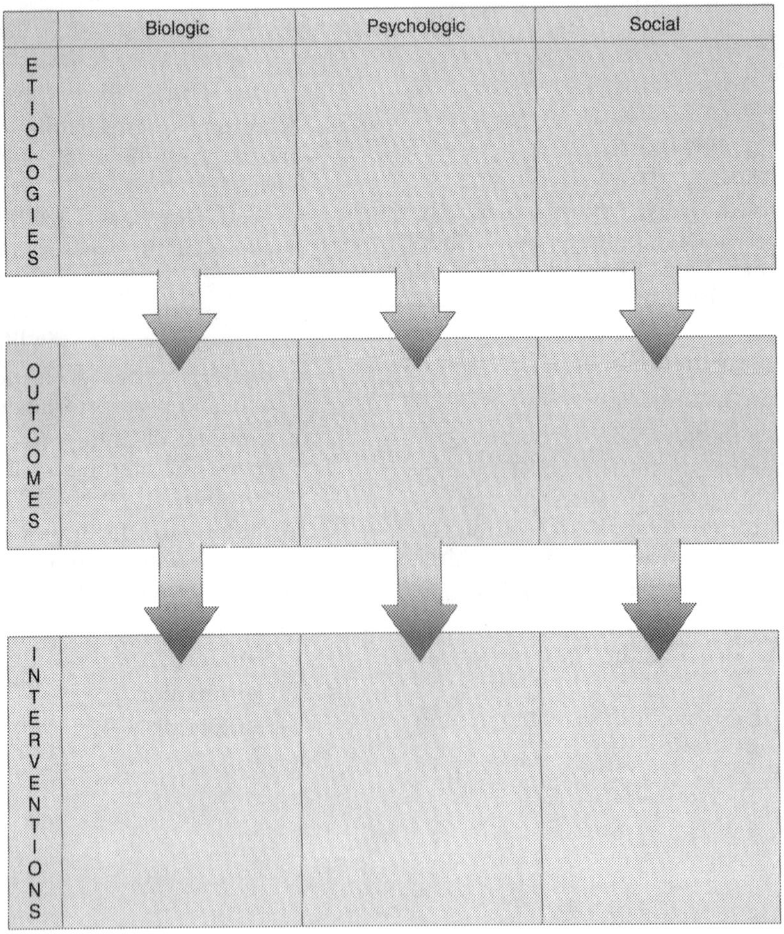

22 ▪ *Substance abuse disorders*

CHAPTER HIGHLIGHTS

Chapter 22 explores substance abuse disorders. It examines the different terms used to describe behaviors with substance use, epidemiologic aspects, possible etiologic theories of causation, and types of substance abuse. The chapter reviews important clinical issues for the nurse and substance abuse treatment interventions and programs. It addresses nursing management for the patient with substance abuse and current professional, social, and political issues related to substance abuse, including the role of the addictions and chemical dependency within nursing.

Chapter 22 key points include the following:

- The DSM IV classifies substance abuse disorders related to the following substances—alcohol, cocaine, amphetamines and other stimulants, cannabis, hallucinogens, phencyclidine, opiates, sedative-hypnotics/anxiolytics, inhalants, nicotine, and caffeine.
- Substance use refers to using substances within the bounds of socially acceptable circumstances and behavior without posing any harm or risk to the individual or others.
- Methadone maintenance treatment, a form of treatment for opiate abusers, involves giving a substitute drug—methadone—in lower, controlled dosages. This helps to satisfy the individual's intense drug craving and counteract the debilitating withdrawal symptoms. Other rehabilitative therapies are used in conjunction with methadone treatment to over addictive behaviors.
- Sedation, reduced memory and concentration, and euphoria indicate opiate intoxication while abdominal cramps, runny nose and eyes, diaphoresis, and insomnia indicate opiate withdrawal.
- Codependency, a maladaptive coping pattern from prolonged exposure to dysfunctional family dynamics associated with active alcohol or drug dependence, is characterized by boundary distortions, poor relationship and friendship skills, compulsive and obsessive behaviors, inappropriate anger, sexual maladjustment, and resistance to change.
- Twelve-step programs, social skills groups, psychoeducational groups, group therapy, and individual and family therapies have been effective in substance abuse treatment.
- Denial of substance abuse problems can be exhibited by attempts to rationalize the substance use, minimize the harmful results, deflect attention from one's own problem, or blame childhood experiences. A non-confrontational approach is crucial.
- Substance abuse programs need to address cultural differences and issues, being responsive to those differences and the specialized needs of cultural and ethnic groups.
- Many social and political ramifications are associated with substance abuse.

STUDENT ACTIVITIES

Labeling

For each concept associated with specific etiologic theories listed below, place the letter of the statement in the correct circle on the biopsychosocial illustration.

a. Affiliation with peer drug use
b. Susceptibility increased by certain personality traits
c. Dysfunctional family dynamics
d. Children of alcoholics with a three to four times greater risk for alcoholism

e. Excessive dependency needs
f. Lack of acetaldehyde dehydrogenase and monoamine oxidase

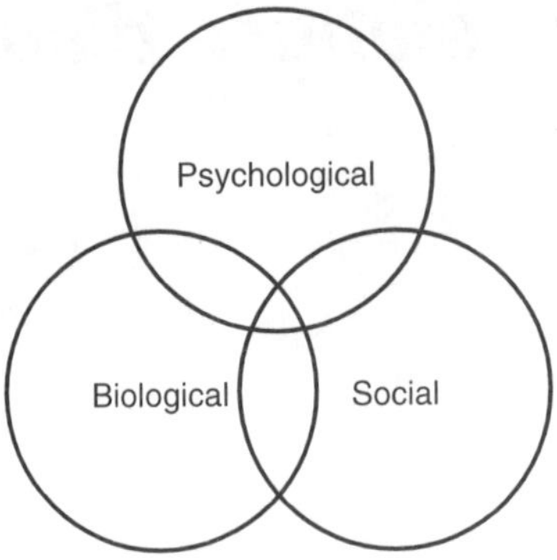

Matching

Place the letter of the description in the righthand column next to the correct term in the lefthand column.

_______ 1. Abuse
_______ 2. Tolerance
_______ 3. Korsakoff's psychosis
_______ 4. Inhalants
_______ 5. Wernicke's syndrome
_______ 6. Dependence
_______ 7. Addiction
_______ 8. Methadone
_______ 9. Hallucinogen
_______ 10. Codependence

a. Reversible alcohol-induced amnesic disorder secondary to thiamine deficiency
b. Severe psychological behavioral dependence on a substance
c. Serotonin agonist producing euphoria or dysphoria
d. Drug used to treat opiate addiction
e. Maladaptive coping pattern of those closely related to the abuser
f. Use of substance for purposes of intoxication
g. Disorder characterized by loss of recent memory and confabulation
h. Volatile substance causing central nervous system depression
i. Need for increased amounts of substance to achieve the same results
j. Continuing use of substance despite adverse consequences to one's well being

Multiple choice

Circle the option that best answers the question.

1. A patient is admitted to the emergency department with a blood alcohol level of 0.10 percent mg. When assessing this patient, the nurse would expect to find which of the following?
   a. Stupor
   b. Ataxia
   c. Incoordination
   d. Emotional lability

2. A patient is admitted to the inpatient psychiatric unit for alcohol detoxification on Sunday. His history reveals twelve years of heavy alcohol intake. His last drink was 24 hours ago. When planning care for this patient, the nurse would anticipate that delirium tremens would most likely occur on which of the following days?
   a. Today (Sunday)
   b. Monday
   c. Thursday
   d. Friday

3. A physician orders disulfiram for a patient with alcohol dependence. Which of the following statements by the patient indicates a need for additional teaching?
   a. "I'll take my over-the-counter cough syrup if I get a cold."
   b. " I'll take the medication at bedtime if it makes me sleepy."
   c. "I'll expect to have a metallic taste in mouth until I'm off the drug."
   d. "I'll continue going to my group therapy meetings."
4. A patient states that he uses free base cocaine. The nurse understands that the patient does which of the following?
   a. Inhales it
   b. Injects it intravenously
   c. Drinks it
   d. Smokes it
5. A patient admitted for the treatment of cocaine intoxication admits to using cocaine in increasing doses. Following admission, the patient sleeps for approximately 16 hours. The nurse understands that this is occurring because of which of the following?
   a. Increased level of prolactin
   b. Depletion of norepinephrine
   c. Serotonin excess
   d. Depletion of dopamine
6. A patient with a history of substance abuse comes to the clinic exhibiting euphoria, sedation, constricted pupils, and difficulty concentrating. Based on these findings, the nurse determines that the patient has used which of the following?
   a. Cocaine
   b. Phencyclidine
   c. Heroin
   d. LSD
7. When interacting with a patient who is hostile and belittling, the nurse becomes frightened and openly expresses anger at the patient's behavior. The nurse is exhibiting which of the following?
   a. Codependence
   b. Denial
   c. Projection
   d. Countertransference
8. The nurse is using motivational interviewing with a patient who is denying a substance abuse problem. When using this technique, the nurse focuses on which of the following?
   a. Confronting the patient's denial openly and forcefully
   b. Telling the patient that he has a problem with substance abuse
   c. Helping the patient make personal choices to gain control
   d. Encouraging the patient to label himself as having an addiction
9. When interviewing the family members of a patient being treated for a substance abuse problem, which of the following behaviors would alert the nurse to the possibility of codependency?
   a. Open expression of thoughts and feelings
   b. Blaming one's self for the family's problems
   c. Being flexible and yet angry
   d. Taking pleasure in self-accomplishments
10. When instituting group therapy for substance abuse problems, the nurse initially plans to focus on which of the following?
   a. Maintaining sobriety
   b. Sustaining abstinence
   c. Coping with early childhood trauma
   d. Using community support services

Critical thinking exercises

1. Using the patient scenario in Nursing Care Plan 22-1 (in the textbook), Jack G., and the chart below, analyze the situation for possible biopsychosocial etiologies and develop appropriate biopsychosocial outcomes and interventions.

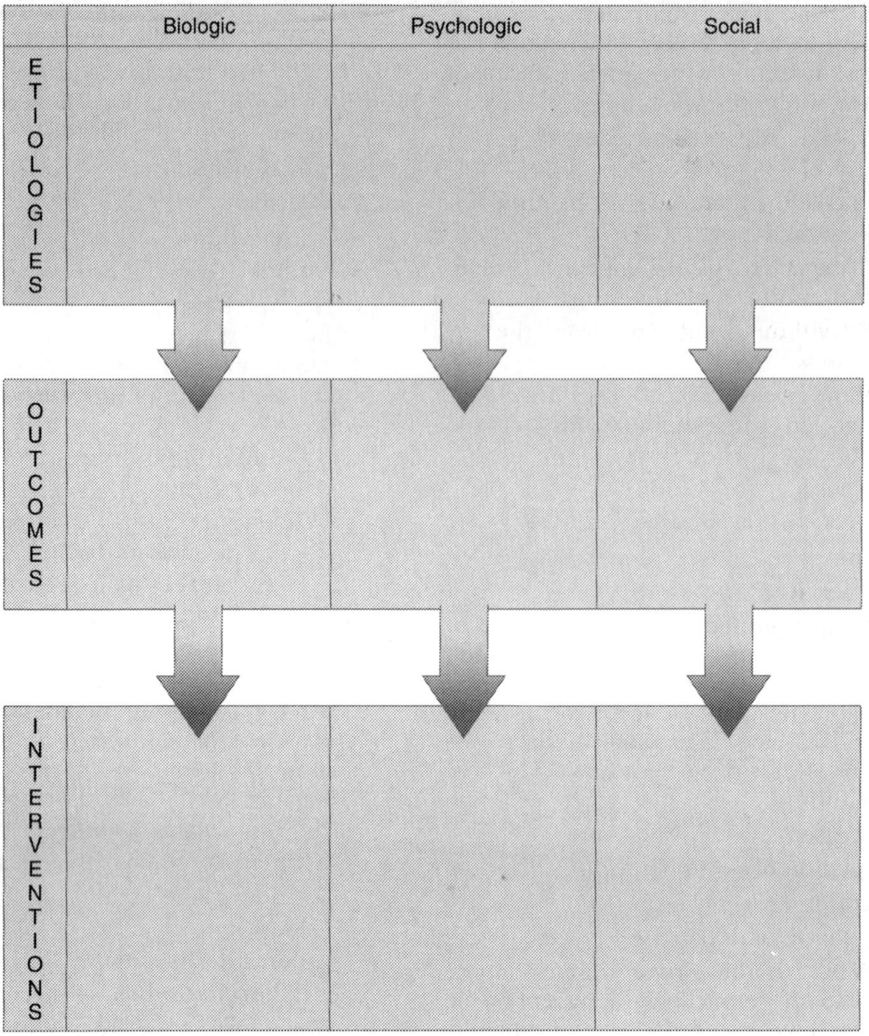

2. A patient suspected of having a cocaine abuse problem states, "I can control my use of cocaine. Besides, I don't use that much. I only use it on the weekends and when I'm on vacation. If you think I use a lot, you should see my friend, Joe. He uses it every day." Develop a therapeutic dialogue, incorporating appropriate therapeutic communication techniques, that addresses this patient's statement. Include a rationale for each technique you used.

3. Explore the Internet for possible organizations and resources for substance abuse. Create a list of these resources for use in a substance abuse teaching program.

4. Attend a community support group meeting for families of patients with substance abuse. Using text box 22-1 (in the textbook), examples of characteristics of codependents, analyze the interactions, providing specific statements or observations that demonstrate codependency in members of the group.

5. A nurse working on your unit has been coming to work late, off and on for the past month. On her arrival to the unit this evening, you notice that the nurse is swaying from side to side when walking, her breath smells of alcohol, and her speech is slightly slurred.
   a. How should you react?

   b. What are your ethical and legal responsibilities to:
      —This nurse

      —The patients

      —Your fellow coworkers

      —The facility

23 ▪ *Sleep disorders*

CHAPTER HIGHLIGHTS

Chapter 23 explores the primary sleep disorders of dyssomnias and parasomnias. It reviews the biologic basis and neurobiologic basis for sleep, biologic measurements of sleep factors, both internal and external, affecting sleep and comorbidity with other psychiatric disorders. This chapter examines the types of dyssomnias including primary insomnia, hypersomnia, narcolepsy, breathing related and circadian rhythm sleep disorders, and parasomnias, such as nightmares, sleep terror, and sleepwalking disorders. Applying the nursing process with integration of the biopsychosocial framework, this chapter describes the nursing management of the patient with a sleep disorder.

Chapter 23 key points include the following:

- Many body systems follow a circadian rhythm, the 24 hours normal sleep-wake cycle.
- Neurochemical activity throughout the CNS is the major mechanism that controls changes in sleep and wakefulness.
- Polysomnography, clinical testing including electroencephalogram, electromyogram, electrooculogram, and measures of oral-nasal airflow, respiratory effort and oxyhemoglobin saturation, describes a person's sleep architecture and any abnormalities occurring during sleep.
- Primary sleep disorders, not the result of another mental or medical disorder or induced by a substance, are ongoing disruptions of normal waking and sleeping patterns, subdivided into dyssomnias and parasomnias.
- Primary insomnia, characterized by either difficulty falling asleep or staying asleep, involves behaviors perpetuating this abnormal sleep pattern. Often precipitated by stress or trauma, sleep preventing association and behaviors develop long after the crisis or stressful situation has passed.
- Obstructive sleep apnea (OSA) syndrome, a commonly diagnosed breathing-related sleep disorder, is characterized by excessive snoring during sleep and episodes of sleep apnea, disrupting sleep and causing daytime sleepiness.
- Somatic interventions for OSA syndrome include nasal CPAP, a surgical treatment that includes vulopalatopharyngoplasty to reconfigure the upper airway.
- Parasomnias, characterized by abnormal physiologic or behavioral events occurring during sleep or transition from sleep to wakefulness, include nightmare, sleep terror, and sleepwalking disorders. These disorders cause unrestful sleep, possibly jeopardizing daytime activities because of excessive sleepiness, poor concentration, and irritability.
- A thorough sleep history, including details of the sleep complaint, current and previous sleeping patterns, medical problems, current medications and life events, and emotional and mental status.
- Nursing interventions focus on education about sleep hygiene, relaxation exercises, and sleep-inducing activities, nutritional counseling regarding what to avoid, and family and friends respecting and encouraging new sleep habits for the patient.

STUDENT ACTIVITIES

Fill in the blanks

Read each statement carefully and place the correct answer in the space(s) provided.

1. The sleep-wake cycle runs in a ________________ rhythm.
2. Wakefulness is maintained by the ____________ in the brain.

3. The predictable pattern of the timing, amount, and distribution of REM and NREM stages during a night's sleep is referred to as ________________.
4. Delta sleep occurs during stages ________ and ________ of NREM sleep.
5. A newborn typically needs approximately ________ hours of sleep each day.
6. A bright light or sunlight is called a ________________.
7. ________ are characterized by disturbances in the amount, quality, or timing of sleep.
8. The hallmark symptom of primary insomnia is the patient's intense focus and anxiety about not being able to ________________ or ________________.
9. ________ is a technique used when the bedroom no longer provides cues for sleep.
10. Narcolepsy includes the tetrad of symptoms of ________, ________, ________, and ________.
11. In children with OSA, ________________ is often the first sign.
12. ________ is a natural substance promoted to reset the circadian clock.
13. Nightmare disorder occurs almost exclusively during ________ sleep.
14. ________ most often happens during the first third of the night.

Multiple choice

Circle the option that best answers the question.

1. Which of the following behaviors would the nurse identify as characteristic of the sleep patterns of a patient experiencing alcohol withdrawal?
   a. Pleasant nondisturbing dreams
   b. Dramatic increase in the number of hours spent sleeping
   c. Fragmented sleep with nightmares
   d. Continuation of the same pattern as when patient was drinking
2. When reviewing the results of polysomnography for the patient with primary insomnia, what would the nurse expect to find?
   a. Increased stage 2 sleep
   b. Poor sleep continuity
   c. Decreased EEG alpha activity
   d. Increased slow wave sleep
3. The nurse instructs the patient with primary insomnia to avoid watching television and eating in the bedroom. The nurse is instructing the patient in which of the following techniques?
   a. Sleep restriction
   b. Relaxation training
   c. Attention focusing
   d. Stimulus control
4. A patient diagnosed with narcolepsy also exhibits bilateral loss of muscle tone triggered by laughing. The nurse identifies this symptom as:
   a. Cataplexy
   b. Hypnagogic hallucinations
   c. Sleep paralysis
   d. Paradoxical reaction
5. The physician orders zolpidem (Ambien) for the treatment of a patient's insomnia. The nurse understands that this drug affects which of the following neurotransmitters?
   a. Dopamine
   b. GABA
   c. Serotonin
   d. Norepinephrine
6. During assessment, which of the following behaviors reported by a patient might alert the nurse to problems sleeping?
   a. Going to bed at the same time each night
   b. Exercising six to seven hours before bedtime
   c. Drinking a cup of tea before bedtime
   d. Keeping the bedroom temperature cool
7. The wife of a patient reports that the patient abruptly sits up at night in bed screaming in fear and panic. She states, "I try to wake him up, but I really can't. When he awakens the next morning, he doesn't remember the episode." The nurse identifies this as which of the following?
   a. Sleep-terror disorder
   b. Sleepwalking disorder
   c. Circadian rhythm sleep disorder
   d. Nightmare disorder

Self-exploration

1. Complete the self assessment questionnaire below. Score your responses and evaluate them. Are you a "lark" or an "owl." Do you agree with this? Please explain why or why not.

<u>The final questionnaire</u>

Instructions:

1. Please read each question very carefully before answering.
2. Answer ALL questions.
3. Answer questions in numerical order.
4. Each question should be answered independently of others. Do NOT go back and check your answers.
5. All questions have a selection of answers. For each question place a cross alongside ONE answer only. Some questions have a scale instead of a selection of answers. Place a cross at the appropriate point along the scale.

<u>The Questionnaire, with scores for each choice</u>

1. Considering only your own "feeling best" rhythm, at what time would you get up if you were entirely free to plan your day?

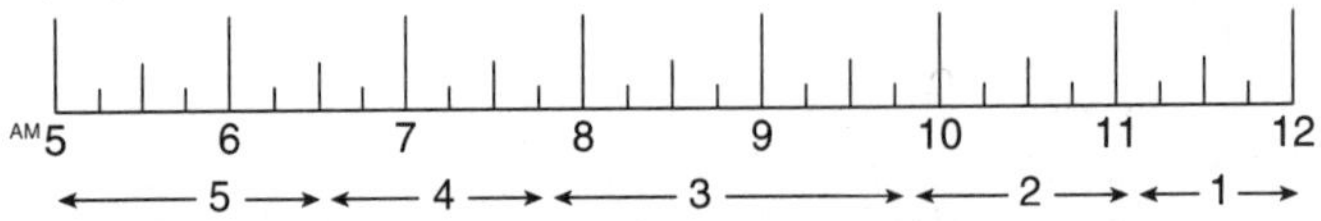

2. Considering only your own "feeling best" rhythm, at what time would you go to bed if you were entirely free to plan your evening?

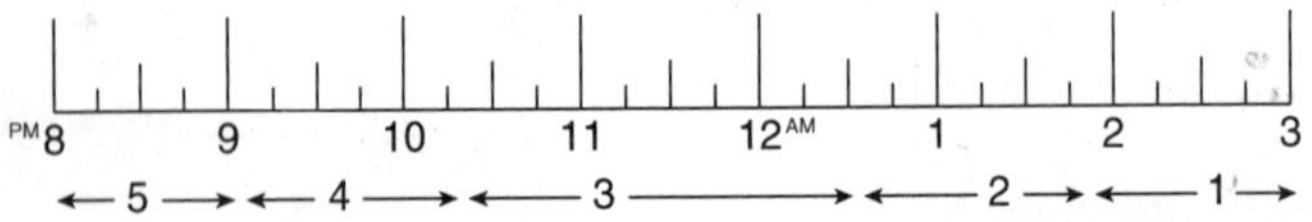

3. If there is a specific time at which you have to get up in the morning, to what extent are you dependent on being woken by an alarm clock?

Not at all dependent...	☐	4
Slightly dependent.....	☐	3
Fairly dependent.......	☐	2
Very dependent.........	☐	1

4. Assuming adequate environmental conditions, how easy do you find getting up in the morning?

Not at all easy..........	☐	1
Not very easy...........	☐	2
Fairly easy...............	☐	3
Very easy................	☐	4

5. How alert do you feel during the first half hour after having woken in the morning?

Not at all alert...........	☐	1
Slightly alert.............	☐	2
Fairly alert...............	☐	3
Very alert.................	☐	4

6. How is your appetite during the first half-hour after having woken in the morning?

Very poor.................	☐	1
Fairly poor...............	☐	2
Fairly good...............	☐	3
Very good................	☐	4

7. During the first half-hour after having woken in the morning, how tired do you feel?

Very tired..........................	☐	1
Fairly tired..........................	☐	2
Fairly refreshed....................	☐	3
Very refreshed.....................	☐	4

8. When you have no commitment the next day, at what time do you go to bed compared to your usual bedtime?

Seldom or never later...........	☐	1
Less than one hour later......	☐	2
1–2 hours later..................	☐	3
More than 2 hours later.........	☐	4

9. You have decided to engage in some physical exercise. A friend suggests that you do this one hour twice a week and the best time for him is between 7:00–8:00AM. Bearing in mind nothing else but your own "feeling best" rhythm how do you think you would perform?

Would be on good form........	☐	1
Would be on reasonable form	☐	2
Would be difficult................	☐	3
Would find it very difficult......	☐	4

10. At what time in the evening do you feel tired and as a result in need of sleep?

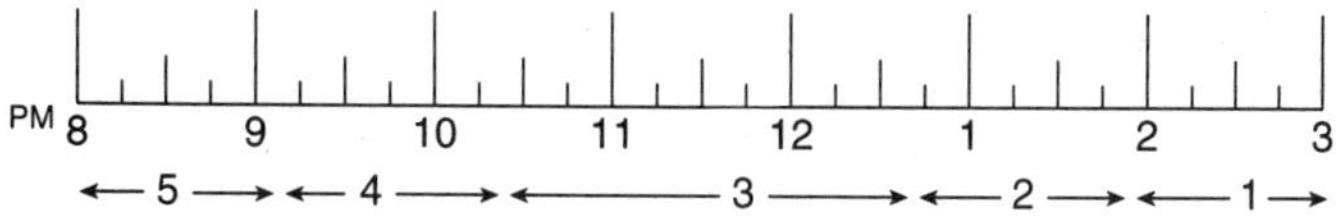

11. You wish to be at your peak performance for a feat which you know is going to be mentally exhausting and lasting for two hours. You are entirely free to plan your day and considering only your own "feeling beat" rhythm which would you choose?

8:00–10:00 AM..................	☐	6
11:00 AM–1:00 PM............	☐	4
3:00–5:00 PM.....................	☐	2
7:00–9:00 PM....................	☐	0

12. If you went to bed at 11:00 PM at what level of tiredness would you be?

Not at all tired......................	☐	0
A little tired...........................	☐	2
Fairly tired............................	☐	3
Very tired..............................	☐	5

13. For some reason you have gone to bed several hours later than usual, but there is no need to get up at any particular time the next morning. Which ONE of the following events are you most likely to experience?

Will wake up at usual time and will NOT fall asleep	☐	4
Will wake up at usual time and will doze thereafter	☐	3
Will wake up at usual time but will fall asleep again	☐	2
Will NOT wake up untill later than usual	☐	1

14. One night you have to remain awake between 4:00–5:00AM in order to carry out a night watch. You have no commitments the next day. Which ONE of the following alternatives will suit you best?

Would NOT go to bed until watch was over	☐	1
Would take a nap before and sleep after	☐	2
Would take a good sleep before and nap after	☐	3
Would take ALL sleep before watch	☐	4

15. You have to do two hours of hard physical work. You are entirely free to plan your day and considfering only your own "feeling best" rhythm which ONE of the following times would you choose?

8:00–10:00 AM....................	☐	4
11:00 AM–1:00 PM.............	☐	3
3:00–5:00 PM.....................	☐	2
7:00–9:00 PM.....................	☐	1

16. You have decided to engage in hard physical exercise. A friend suggests that you do this for one hour twice a week and the best time for him is between 10:00–11:00 PM. Bearing in mind nothing else but your own "feeling best" rhythm how well do you think you would perform?

Would be on good form........	☐	4
Would be on reasonable form	☐	3
Would find it difficult............	☐	2
Would find it very difficult......	☐	1

17. Suppose that you can choose your own work hour. Assume that you worked a FIVE hour day (including breaks) and that your job was interesting and paid by results. Which FIVE CONSECUTIVE HOURS would you select?

12 1 2 3 4 5 6 7 8 9 10 11 12 1 2 3 4 5 6 7 8 9 10 11 12

MIDNIGHT NOON MIDNIGHT

← 1 → ← 5 → ←4→ ← 3 → ← 2 → ← 1 →

18. At what time of the day do you think that you reach your "feeling best" peak?

12 1 2 3 4 5 6 7 8 9 10 11 12 1 2 3 4 5 6 7 8 9 10 11 12

MIDNIGHT NOON MIDNIGHT

— 1 → ← 5 → ← 4 → ← 3 → ← 2 → ← 1 →

19. One hears about "morning" and "evening" types of people. Which ONE of these types do you consider yourself to be?

Definitely a "morning" type	☐	6
Rather more a "morning" than an "evening" type	☐	4
Rather more an "evening" than a "morning" type	☐	2
Definitely an "evening" type	☐	0

<u>Scoring</u> For questions 3, 4, 5, 6, 7, 8, 9, 11, 12, 13, 14, 15, 16 and 19, the appropriate score for each response is displayed beside the answer box.

For questions 1, 2, 10 and 18, the cross made along each scale is referred to the appropriate score value range below the scale.

For question 17 the most extreme cross on the right hand side is taken as the reference point and the appropriate score value range below this point is taken.

The scores are added together and the sum converted into a five point Morningness-Eveningness scale:

	Score
Definitely Morning Type	70–86
Moderately Morning Type	59–69
Neither Type	42–58
Moderately Evening Type	31–41
Definitely Evening Type	16–30

2. After reviewing the routine that you go through before going to bed at night, analyze it for measures that both promote sleep or might interfere with it. Postulate alternative measures for those determined as interferences.

Critical thinking exercises

1. An obese middle-aged male is brought to the facility for evaluation of his snoring. His wife states, "He snores so loud sometimes I have to sleep in another room with the door closed. It really scares me because when he snores, he often stops breathing for a few seconds." The patient is scheduled for polysomonography.
   a. Develop a teaching plan for this patient to prepare him for the procedure. A diagnosis of OSA syndrome is made and the patient is to receive nasal CPAP at home. You are the nurse assigned to visit the patient at home.
   b. Create a patient instruction sheet that reflects the teaching plan about his disorder and the use of CPAP for this patient and his wife.
2. Using the questions listed in text box 23-5 (in the textbook), Sleep Assessment Questions, assess an assigned patient's sleep. What conclusions can you draw from your assessment?
3. Using the patient scenario presented in Nursing Care Plan 23-1 (in the textbook), Matthew, and the chart below, analyze the situation for possible biopsychosocial etiologies, and develop appropriate biopsychosocial outcomes and interventions.

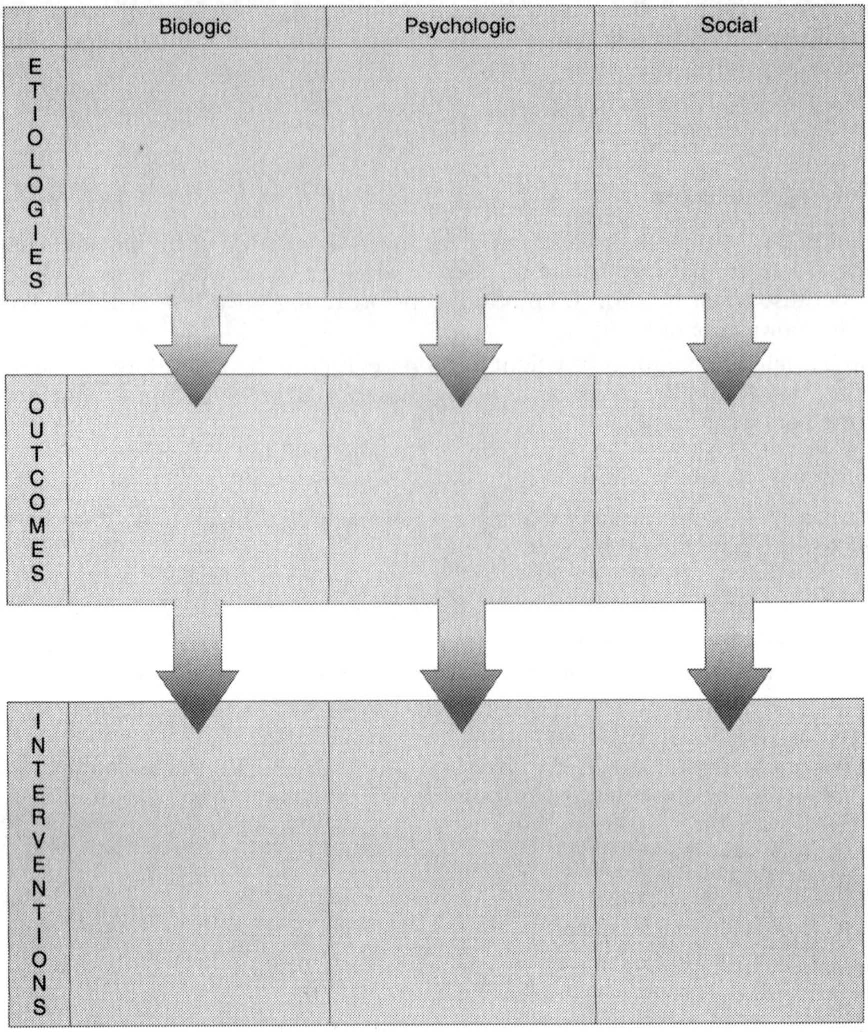

4. Using the clinical vignette presented in text box 23-1 (in the textbook), Jim, develop an appropriate plan of care that addresses his priority needs.

5. Interview a nurse who works the night shift on a permanent basis and a nurse who works rotating shifts. Compare and contrast their sleep patterns, circadian rhythms, and risk for sleep disorders.

24 ▪ *Sexual disorders*

CHAPTER HIGHLIGHTS

Chapter 24 explores sexual disorders. It reviews sexual development from infancy through death and human sexual response. This chapter examines various sexual disorders including orgasmic disorders, sexual arousal disorders and other sexual disorders, such as those involving desire and pain and those caused by a general medical condition, dysfunction resulting from substances, paraphilias, and gender identity disorders. Applying the nursing process with integration of the biopsychosocial framework, this chapter describes the nursing management of a patient with either a female orgasmic disorder or a male erectile disorder.

Chapter 24 key points include the following:

- Sexuality is a basic dimension of every individual's personality, undergoing periods of growth and development and influenced by biologic and psychosocial factors.
- People can maintain their sexuality throughout their lifetime.
- Sexual response consists of four phases—desire, excitement, orgasm, and resolution. Sexual disorders are characterized by a change in sexual desire and sexual response that causes emotional and interpersonal distress.
- Female orgasmic disorder is one of the most common disorders affecting erectile dysfunction; premature ejaculation is most common in men.
- Sexual history is a key part of the nursing assessment. A nurse needs to be comfortable with his or her own sexuality to collect meaningful assessment data.
- Counseling, education, and referral to sex therapists are important interventions for a person with a sexual dysfunction.
- Various medications can negatively affect the sexual response cycle. Education about possible medication side effects and sexual experiences are important for maintaining health.
- Paraphilias are rarely diagnosed but may be more prevalent than what is presented.
- Gender identity disorders occur when the individual is uncomfortable with assigned sex or gender role.

STUDENT ACTIVITIES

Word unscramble

Below is a list of scrambled words. Unscramble each word and place it in the appropriate space next to its definition.

dngere ytitnedi	msgroa
teihfsmis	yspredauian
enopmasue	hapapiiasrl
ishibioexitnm	xcemneitet

______________ 1. The use of an object for sexual arousal.

______________ 2. Sexual behaviors most persons would define as deviant, unusual, or perverse.

______________ 3. The internal sense of one's self as male or female.

______________ 4. Gradual cessation of menstruation and ovulation ending reproductive capacity.

______________ 5. Pain during intercourse.

______________ 6. Phase of sexual response involving semen ejaculation.

______________ 7. State of mounting sexual tension characterized by vasoconstriction and myotonia.

______________ 8. Exposure of one's genitals to strangers.

Labeling

On the sexual response event line below, place the letter of the event in the correct phase.

a. Prostate contraction
b. Involuntary pelvic thrusting
c. Lubrication from vaginal walls
d. Nipple erection
e. Subsiding of vasocongestion
f. Penile erection
g. Semen ejaculation
h. Uterine elevation complete
i. Gradual return of vaginal color
j. Increased vaginal length

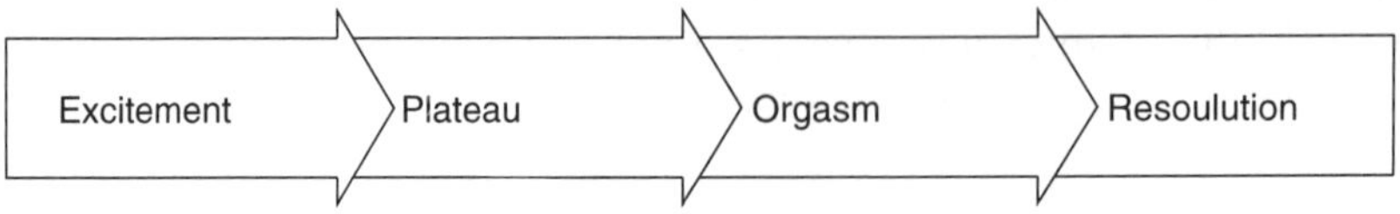

Multiple choice

Circle the option that best answers the question.

1. In teaching a group of students about sexual development, the instructor describes biosexual identity. The instructor correctly states that it is which of the following?
   a. Outward expression of one's gender
   b. Internal sense of one's self as male or female
   c. Individual's feelings of sexual attraction
   d. Anatomic and physiologic state of male or female

2. The nurse is to conduct a health education class for a group of middle-aged males. When preparing for this class, the nurse makes sure to address male sexual changes, including which of the following?
   a. Increased viability of sperm
   b. More firm erections
   c. Decreased testosterone production
   d. Increase in testicular size

3. When counseling an older couple about sexual function, the nurse advises the couple that:
   a. Erections usually can be maintained for a longer period of time
   b. Women need less time to adequately lubricate the vagina
   c. Less direct stimulation is needed for an erection
   d. Loss of sexual desire is inevitable

4. The sex therapist instructs the couple in sensate focus therapy. Which of the following correctly describes this technique?
   a. Exercises used to strengthen the pubococcygeal muscles
   b. Learning and communicating about what each finds arousing
   c. Using masturbation to produce orgasm
   d. Employing fantasies to achieve arousal

5. When obtaining a patient's sexual history, the nurse should do which of the following?
   a. Allow the patient to raise the topic
   b. Interview the couple together about their problems
   c. Respect the patient's refusal to answer a question
   d. Phrase questions to elicit a yes or no answer

6. A patient is diagnosed with male orgasmic disorder and the physician orders intracavernosal pharmacotherapy. When developing a teaching plan, the nurse demonstrates understanding of this treatment by describing it as which of the following?
   a. Suppository insert into the urethra
   b. Aphrodisiac taken to stimulate erection
   c. Surgical implantation of drugs via a prosthesis
   d. Injection of medication into the penis

7. When developing a plan of care for a woman with dyspareunia, the nurse remembers that this condition is most commonly the result of which of the following?
   a. Decreased lubrication
   b. Involuntary muscle spasm
   c. Localized infection
   d. Malignancy

8. When assessing a patient's sexual history, the patient reports becoming sexually aroused when his genitals rub against the breasts of another person who didn't consent to be touched. The nurse identifies this as which of the following?
   a. Fetishism
   b. Frotteurism
   c. Sexual masochism
   d. Sexual sadism

Critical thinking exercises

1. Using the patient scenario presented in Nursing Care Plan 24-1 (in the textbook), Alice Davidson, and the chart below, analyze the situation for possible biopsychosocial etiologies and develop appropriate biopsychosocial outcomes and interventions.

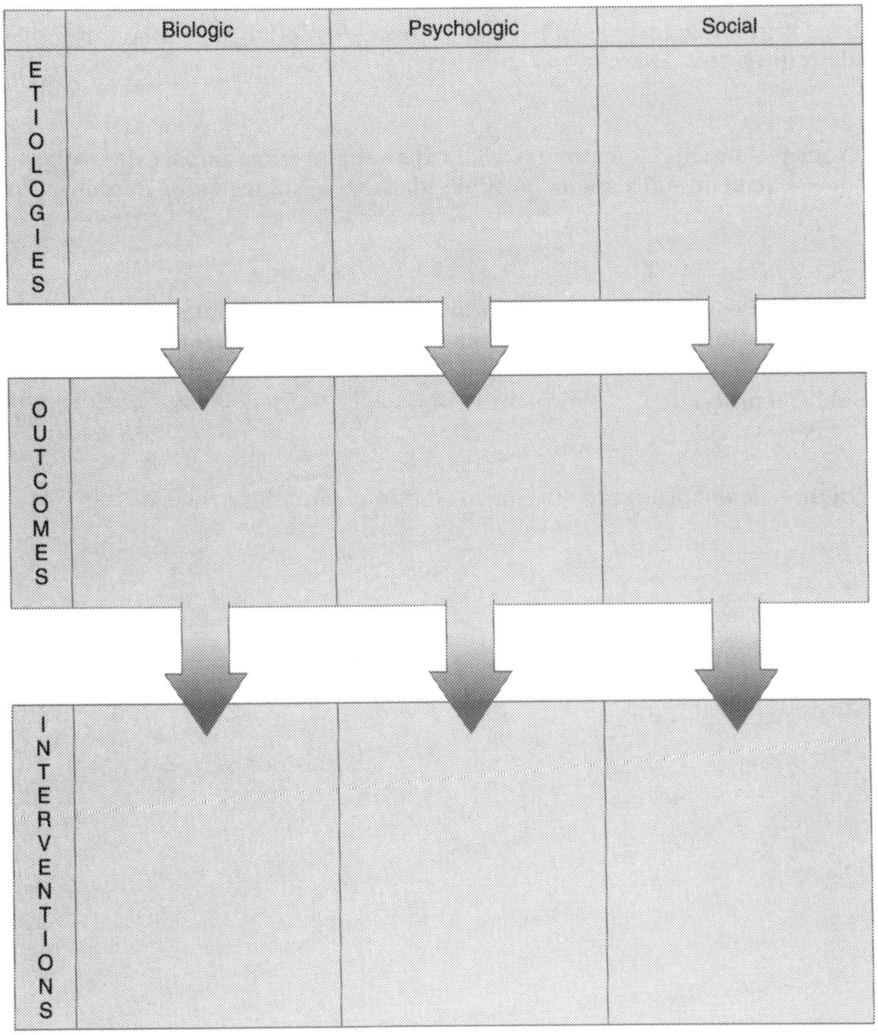

2. Imagine if you were asked to teach a health promotion class on sexuality to a group of young adult couples in their early twenties. The group includes both heterosexual and homosexual couples.
   a. How would you approach this task?

b. What information would you plan to include?

c. Develop a teaching plan that would meet the needs of this group. Include any suggestions for audiovisual aids and handouts for the class.

3. As part of a class assignment, you are to choose another classmate as a partner and interview each other to obtain a sexual history.

   a. What feelings did you experience when you were the interviewer? Explore these feelings as they related to a specific topic.

   b. What feelings did you experience when you were the one being interviewed? Explore these feelings as they relate to a specific topic.

   c. At any time, were these feelings noticeable to your partner? If so, explain how or what it was that made your partner aware of your feelings.

   d. Analyze your feelings and behaviors to determine the possible impact they might have if the partner was a patient and explore possible alternative strategies to minimize any negative impact.

5. A patient's husband comes to the clinic. During the course of the interview, the husband states, "My wife doesn't love me any more. She never wants to have sex with me. When she does, I feel like she's just doing it to placate me. I've tried everything."

   a. How would you proceed?

   b. Develop a therapeutic dialogue with this patient to explore his concerns.

UNIT FIVE
Care of special populations

25 ▪ *Mental health promotion with children and adolescents*

CHAPTER HIGHLIGHTS

Chapter 25 provides a framework for assessing and promoting the mental health of children and adolescents. It explores the ways that young people cope with common life stressors, identifies risk factors for psychopathology, and provides guidelines for mental health promotion and risk reduction.

Chapter 25 key points include the following:

- Nurses working with children and adolescents are in a key position to identify risk and protective factors for psychopathology and to intervene for risk reduction.
- Knowledge of normal development can help nurses educate parents about their children's behaviors, better understand their children's reactions to stress, and decide when intervention is needed.
- If trauma or neglect disrupt normal childhood biologic maturation, developmental delays, some with irreversible effects, can occur.
- A difficult temperament in childhood has been correlated with the development of various forms of psychopathology.
- Language development depends on a complex interaction between physical maturation, physical and neuromuscular maturation of the head and neck, hearing ability, cognitive abilities, exposure to language, educational stimulation, and emotional well- being.
- The quality of the child and parent emotional bond is an important determinant of the success of later relationships.
- Disruption in attachments, such as out-of-home placement or adoption, may lead to difficulties in forming close relationships with new parents or trusting others.
- Cognitive, moral, psychosexual, and psychosocial developmental theories can serve as a framework for understanding a child's view of the world and key tasks of each developmental period.
- Assessment methods need to be adapted to the needs of the child and family based on their culture and present problems.
- Children who experience major losses have been shown to be at risk for developing psychopathology.
- Sibling relationships have a significant impact on personality. If positive, they can be a protective factor against the development of psychopathology.
- Childhood and adolescent medical problems, when illness leads to regression or a lack of full participation in activities, may cause psychological problems.
- Adolescents, in their striving for identity and independence, may participate in high-risk activities, creating a risk for mental health problems.

- Conditions such as poverty, homelessness, abuse, neglect, and parental alcoholism may undermine the child's ability to achieve normal developmental gains, thus making them more vulnerable for emotional and behavioral problems.
- Family support services and early intervention programs aim to prevent the removal of the abused or neglected child from the family, and maintain a strong nurturing family system.
- Psychoeducational approaches, such as training, group experiences, and bibliotherapy, provide children and their families with the information and skills to foster their own mental health.
- The nurse promotes mental health by acting as an advocate, partner, and educator to empower families to identify and meet their own needs.

STUDENT ACTIVITIES

Matching

Place the letter of the description in the right hand column next to the correct term in the lefthand column.

_______ 1. Animism
_______ 2. Maturation
_______ 3. Assortive mating
_______ 4. Plasticity
_______ 5. Conservation
_______ 6. Egocentrism
_______ 7. Moral idealism
_______ 8. Temperament
_______ 9. Integration
_______ 10. Object permanence

a. Selection of partner with similar genetically linked traits
b. Person's characteristic intensity, rhythmicity, adaptability, and energy expenditure
c. Awareness of the existence of a person when not physically present
d. View of the world as revolving around one's self
e. Use of passionate philosophical positions on controversial issues
f. Efficient communication through cellular mechanisms for information synthesis
g. Belief that inanimate objects are alive
h. Ability to take over function of damaged area
i. Awareness that quantity remains the same despite a change in shape
j. Orderly sequence of biologic and genetic growth interacting and dependent on the environment

Self-exploration

1. Think back on a time when you were younger and experienced the loss of a significant person or object.
   a. How did this loss make you feel?

   b. How did you react to this loss?

   c. Would your reaction be different today or similar to what it was then? Explain how.

2. Imagine that you are assigned to care for a family and their child who is a suspected victim of physical abuse.
   a. Identify your feelings related to this child and family.

   b. Propose appropriate strategies to deal with this situation nonjudgmentally.

3. Review your relationship with your siblings. Evaluate the positive and negative impacts of your relationship with them on your development.

Labeling

On the grid below, shade in the area along the line that correctly corresponds to the age span for the developmental state listed to the left.

	Age in Years								
Developmental Stage	*0*	*2*	*4*	*6*	*8*	*11*	*12*	*14*	*16+*
Preoperational									
Anal									
Conventional									
Initiative vs. Guilt									
Concrete Operations									
Latency									
Sensorimotor									
Industry vs. Inferiority									
Genital									

Multiple choice

Circle the option that best answers the question.

1. Which of the following behaviors would be typical of an 8-year-old child who has experienced the death of a loved one?
   a. Repeated questioning about the person's death
   b. Frequent statements that the person will be coming back
   c. Comfort seeking with his peers
   d. Experimentation with killing insects
2. While assessing a child's development, the nurse places two glasses, one wide and short and one tall and slender, each containing the same amount of water, in front of the child. The nurse asks the child to pick the glass that has more water. The child responds that both glasses are the same. The child is exhibiting which of the following?
   a. Object permanence
   b. Conservation
   c. Egocentrism
   d. Animism
3. An adolescent becomes passionately involved in a local group advocating the legalization of marijuana. The adolescent is exhibiting:
   a. Moral idealism
   b. Postconventional reasoning
   c. Identity
   d. Autonomy
4. Key to assessing an adolescent is the issue of:
   a. Honesty
   b. Clarity
   c. Empathy
   d. Confidentiality
5. During an interview, the nurse asks a child, "If you had three wishes, what would you wish for?" The nurse is attempting to elicit information about which of the following?
   a. Daily life and play
   b. View of self and their world
   c. Thoughts of violence
   d. Mental status

6. Divorced parents of a child come to the clinic for some help with easing their child's transition to the divorce. Which of the following suggestions would be helpful for the parents to institute?
   a. Unstructured visitation schedule
   b. Changes in usual routines
   c. Reinforcement of the reasons for divorce
   d. Consistent limit setting with behavior
7. A 7-year-old child is brought to the emergency room by his mother with a fracture of the humerus from "walking into the door." Upon examination, the nurse also notes some clusters of bruising in various stages of healing on the thighs. History reveals previous fractures of ulna and wrist. When questioned, the mother states, "He's a very active but clumsy child. He's always falling over something." The nurse suspected possible physical abuse. Which of the following would help to confirm the nurse's suspicions?
   a. Crying when the nurse obtains a blood specimen
   b. Withdrawing when the nurse attempts to touch the child
   c. Clinging to the mother during the examination
   d. Child openly reporting incident to the nurse
8. The nurse is involved with an adoptive parents support group. To assist the parents with adjustment, the nurse anticipates that following the initial adjustment and attachment period, the next most common difficult period is:
   a. Preschool
   b. School age
   c. Adolescence
   d. Adulthood
9. During an assessment of a child with alcoholic parents, the child states, "I make sure that my younger brother and sister are washed, dressed, and ready for school every morning. I even make their lunches." The nurse determines that this child is acting in which of the following roles?
   a. Hero
   b. Scapegoat
   c. Mascot
   d. Lost child
10. During an interview, a preschooler states, "I don't like when my mom vacuums the rug. I'm afraid it'll eat me." The nurse interprets this statement as an example of which of the following?
   a. Transitional object
   b. Guilt
   c. Formal operations
   d. Animism

Critical thinking exercises

1. Visit a local homeless shelter in your area. Identify the mental health issues for the children in this shelter and propose various strategies to meet their needs.

2. Interview the parents of an adopted child. Explore their process of adjustment and describe any problems that they have encountered.

3. A 10-year-old child has a history of severe asthma since age 2½ years. During his illness, he has required numerous hospitalizations causing him to miss school frequently. The severity of his asthma also has resulted in curtailing his physical activity, so that he has been rather sedentary and has not experienced typical peer relationships. Although his asthma is manageable at present, the parents come to you for guidance. Develop a plan of care that addresses the needs of the child and his family that will promote optimal development.

4. As part of a class assignment, you are required to observe a support group, such as Al-Anon or Adult Children of Alcoholics (ACOA). Prepare a presentation that describes the group process you observed and the issues addressed.

26 ▪ Care of children and adolescents with psychiatric disorders

CHAPTER HIGHLIGHTS

Chapter 26 explores the major psychiatric disorders encountered with children and adolescents. It focuses on developmental, disruptive behavior, mood and anxiety, and tic disorders, while briefly reviewing other childhood disorders such as elimination disorders and childhood schizophrenia. Applying the nursing process with integration of the biopsychosocial framework, this chapter describes the nursing management for the patient with pervasive developmental disorders and disruptive behavior disorders, specifically attention deficit/hyperactivity disorder (ADHD) and conduct problems.

Chapter 26 key points include the following:

- Improved assessment methods and definitions have resulted in better appreciation for the frequency of psychiatric disorders in children and adolescents. Approximately 12 percent of those under age 18 in the United States have a psychiatric disorder.
- Developmental disorders include mental retardation, pervasive developmental disorders, and specific developmental disorders, such as communication and learning disorders, which are now more frequent in children with other primary psychiatric disorders.
- Childhood psychiatric disorders can be divided into externalizing disorders, such as disruptive behavior disorders (ADHD, oppositional defiant, and conduct disorders) or internalizing disorders, such as depression and anxiety disorders.
- ADHD, the most common childhood disorder affecting boys more often than girls, is defined by the presence of inattention, impulsiveness, and hyperactivity (in most cases). Treatment approaches include medications, parent training, and child behavioral treatment.
- Oppositional defiant disorder is characterized by persistent disobedience, argumentativeness, and tantrums.
- Conduct disorder is characterized by lying, truancy, stealing, and fighting.
- Separation anxiety and obsessive compulsive disorders are relatively frequent anxiety disorders in school-aged children. Treatment includes medications, behavioral therapy, alone or in combination.
- Major depression in children is believed to be similar to that in adults. However, efficacy of antidepressant medications is less well established.
- Tourette's syndrome, a tic disorder, is characterized by motor and phonic tics. Common comorbid conditions include ADHD and obsessive compulsive disorder.
- Childhood schizophrenia is rare in children.
- Elimination disorders, such as encopresis and enuresis, are treated most effectively with behavioral therapy.

STUDENT ACTIVITIES

Word find

Hidden within the following letter grid are key terms from chapter 26, listed below. The terms may be vertical, horizontal, diagonal, or backward. Circle the words as you find them.

Attention
Autism
Conduct disorder
Desensitization
Dyslexia
Echolalia
Encopresis
Enuresis
Hyperactivity
Impulsiveness
Learning disorder
School phobia
Tics

I	N	T	E	R	M	O	D	A	L	S	I	S	M	L	E
Y	C	O	N	D	U	C	T	D	I	S	O	R	D	E	R
T	D	E	V	E	L	O	Y	P	M	E	N	T	E	A	E
A	I	S	I	S	E	R	P	O	C	N	E	O	S	R	T
I	S	T	L	E	N	M	U	H	H	E	C	U	E	N	S
B	N	A	Z	L	O	S	N	B	Y	V	H	R	N	I	B
O	A	T	E	D	I	E	T	I	P	I	O	E	S	N	E
H	I	S	C	I	T	I	X	A	E	S	L	D	I	G	H
P	X	O	R	R	N	T	A	I	R	L	A	I	T	D	A
L	E	N	U	R	E	S	I	S	A	U	L	S	I	I	V
O	L	I	N	G	T	U	E	R	A	P	I	O	Z	S	P
O	S	M	E	N	T	A	D	U	C	M	A	R	A	O	R
H	Y	P	E	R	A	C	T	I	V	I	T	Y	T	R	O
C	D	A	T	T	E	I	N	O	T	I	V	T	I	D	D
S	N	O	I	T	S	T	T	E	R	U	O	T	O	E	E
O	I	T	A	M	C	I	N	U	M	M	O	C	N	R	R

Fill in the blanks

Read each statement carefully and place the correct answer in the space(s) provided.

1. ______________ is below average intelligence accompanied by impaired adaptive functioning.
2. Autism is distinguished by the presence of ________________ and __________________ .
3. Repetitive rocking and hand flapping are examples of ________________________________ .
4. ______________disorders appear more commonly in boys, often running in families with a high occurrence in fathers.
5. The comorbid condition of ________________ disorders is common in children with autism.
6. Children with PDD who are hospitalized require ______________ for successful treatment.
7. The underlying problem for reading disability appears to be a deficit in ________________ .
8. Reading disability is believed to be the result of a problem in the ____________ hemisphere of the brain, while mathematics disorder appears to be a problem in _____________ hemisphere.
9. The ________________ mandates that public school systems provide remedial service in the least restrictive educational setting for those identified with a learning disability.
10. Attention deficit hyperactivity disorder is referred to as an _______________ disorder based on the "acting out" behavior.
11. In ADHD, _____________ functions appear to be deficient.
12. One of the most frequently diagnosed disorders in children in mental health facilities is ____ .
13. Obsessive compulsive disorder in children is frequently accompanied by ______________ and ____________ disorders.
14. Research has postulated that Tourette's syndrome involves some abnormality of ___________ .
15. Encopresis and enuresis are more commonly seen in ______________________________ .

Multiple choice

Circle the option that best answers the question.

1. When assessing a child for the possibility of autism, the nurse would expect to find which of the following?
   a. Close interaction with other children
   b. Flexibility in adhering to routines
   c. Ability to maintain a conversation
   d. Repetitive motor mannerisms
2. When dealing with the parents of a child diagnosed with PDD, which of the following statements by the nurse would be appropriate?
   a. "Use 'time out' as a way to control any aggressive behavior."
   b. "Ignore his head banging, it's just for attention."
   c. "Allow the child to come up with a list of routine activities."
   d. "Encourage the child to talk when he is around others."
3. When assessing the child with communication disorder, the nurse would expect to find which of the following?
   a. Positive self-image
   b. Easily cooperative
   c. Socially isolated
   d. An accompanying reading disability
4. A student is studying for an examination on ADHD. The student requires additional review if the student identifies which of the following as a core symptom?
   a. Hyperactivity
   b. Aggressiveness
   c. Impulsiveness
   d. Inattention
5. The physician orders methylphenidate hydrochloride daily in divided doses for a child with ADHD. The child receives his first dose at 8 A.M. every morning before going to school. When would the school nurse anticipate the possibility of a return of the child's behavior?
   a. 10 A.M.
   b. 11 A.M.
   c. 12 P.M.
   d. 1 P.M.
6. When teaching the parents of a child with ADHD, which of the following statements by the parents would indicate the need for additional teaching?
   a. "We'll make sure to have him complete one task before going on to another one."
   b. "We'll let him do his homework in the kitchen while I'm cooking dinner."
   c. "We'll use simple, clear directions and instructions."
   d. "We'll set up rules with specific times for eating, sleeping, and playing."
7. A child with a conduct disorder is receiving problem-solving therapy. The nurse understands that which of the following will most likely be included?
   a. Event interpretation
   b. Positive reinforcement
   c. Role playing
   d. Therapist modeling
8. A child is diagnosed with school phobia. As part of the treatment, the child is rapidly and forcibly returned to school. The nurse identifies this technique as:
   a. Behavior modification
   b. Aversion therapy
   c. Desensitization
   d. Flooding
9. When evaluating a child for major depressive disorder, it is important for the nurse to keep in mind which of the following?
   a. Children act out their feelings rather than discuss them
   b. Children spontaneously reveal sadness and worthlessness
   c. Pharmacologic treatment with antidepressants is highly effective
   d. The child's functional level is usually unimpaired

Critical thinking exercises

1. Using the patient scenario presented in Nursing Care Plan 26-1 (in the textbook), Jamie, and the chart on page 124, identify possible biopsychosocial etiologies for this patient and develop appropriate biopsychosocial outcomes and interventions.

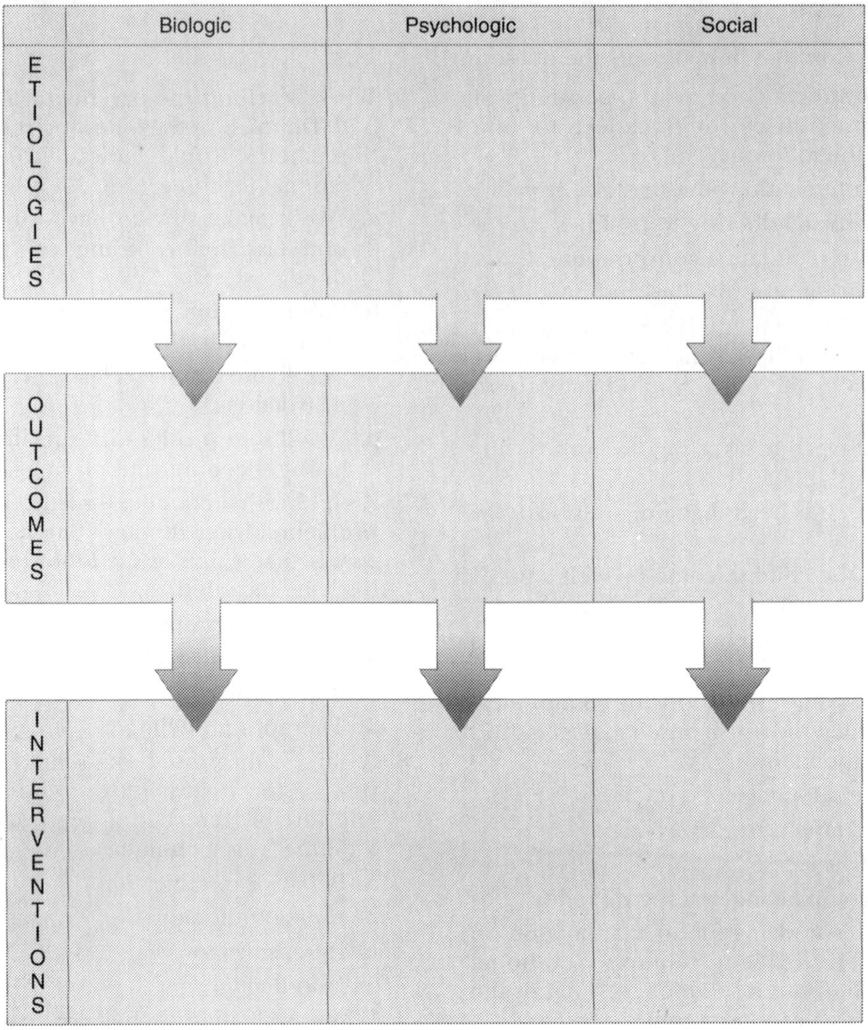

2. A patient diagnosed with ADHD is to receive methylphenidate. Develop a teaching plan for the parents and child, incorporating your knowledge of the disorder and the drug.

3. Review the clinical vignette presented in text box 26-4 (in the textbook), Leon. After analyzing the information, identify Leon's priority nursing diagnoses and develop a plan of care that addresses these priorities. Be sure to integrate possible treatment options into this plan.

4. Review the Education for the Handicapped Act (PL 94-142). Investigate your local public school district to determine how it complies with this mandate.

5. Interview the parents of a child diagnosed with ADHD. Explore their feelings and the impact of the disorder on their family life.

27 ▪ *Biopsychosocial care of the elderly mentally ill*

CHAPTER HIGHLIGHTS

Chapter 27 addresses the biopsychosocial care of the elderly mentally ill population, including psychopharmacologic considerations and residential care. It reviews the mental health problems associated with aging based on neurobiologic changes, psychological aspects, social and cultural issues, and developmental tasks. It explores the assessment of the geriatric mental health patient and interventions for geropsychiatric disorders, such as depression and anxiety, and chronic psychiatric disorders such as schizophrenia.

Chapter 27 key points include the following:

- Ethnicity affects the perception and treatment of elders in their community, distribution of mental disorders, and use of formal and informal health services.
- Normal age-related changes are universal, progressive, decremental, and intrinsic. Sensory function declines and reaction time slows with age. Intelligence and personality remain stable over the life span.
- Medications, depression, poor nutrition, infection, heart and lung disease, thyroid problems, alcohol use, and sensory loss threaten the elder's memory.
- Depression, a major mental health problem for the elderly, is implicated in approximately ⅔ of elder suicides.
- Elderly patients receive antianxiety agents at five times the rate of the general population, even with a lower prevalence of anxiety disorders in this population.
- Little is known about the long-term course of schizophrenia in the elderly.
- Nonpharmacologic interventions, preferred because of the elderly's increased risk for adverse drug reactions, may include reminiscence, life review, pet therapy, music therapy, remotivation, and psychodrama.
- Aging affect all aspects of a drug's pharmacokinetics and also the strength and number of protein-binding sites.
- Assisted living empowers the individual to maintain independence, while providing nursing services and case management within the least restrictive environment.
- Residential care, when necessary, should emphasize family-centered care, while optimizing existing functional capabilities.

STUDENT ACTIVITIES

Matching

Place the letter of the description in the righthand column next to the correct term in the lefthand column.

_______ 1. Memory
_______ 2. Exposure therapy
_______ 3. Reminiscence
_______ 4. Ethnicity
_______ 5. Cognition
_______ 6. Life review
_______ 7. Bereavement
_______ 8. Metabolism
_______ 9. Half-life
_______ 10. Psychodrama

a. Mental process characterized by knowing, thinking, learning, and judging
b. Period of profound grieving after a loss
c. Time to decrease the amount of drug in the body by 50 percent
d. Group role-playing technique used for emotional expression and problem exploration
e. Biotransformation
f. Critical analysis of one's past
g. Information storage system
h. In vivo desensitization
i. Free-flowing spontaneous look at specific events in one's life
j. Variations based on national origin

Self-exploration

1. Imagine that you are a widowed 80-year-old with multiple health problems. You live alone without the support of close family nearby. Your only support is a neighbor, who does your grocery shopping once a week, and a 72-year-friend, who takes you to the doctor and runs errands for you about once or twice a week. Identify the possible problems that you might face and explore possible resolutions.

2. As part of a simulation exercise, you are to play an elderly patient with typical neurobiological changes carrying out activities of daily living. You wear glasses coated with Vaseline to impair your sight, gloves to diminish your sense of touch, cotton in your ears to diminish your hearing, and two different height shoes to simulate gait and joint problems. The simulation lasts a half an hour.
   a. What observations did you note?

   b. What feelings did you experience?

   c. Would this experience change the way you relate to an elderly person? Why or why not?

Multiple choice

Circle the option that best answers the question.

1. When assessing an elderly patient, the nurse would identify which of the following as normal age-related changes?
   a. Delayed reaction time
   b. Impaired consciousness
   c. Memory loss
   d. Decreased taste threshold

2. Based on the studies of the elderly population, which of the following statements is true?
   a. White elders have higher morbidity than minority elders, including African Americans.
   b. African-American elderly have lower rates of depression than other elderly groups.
   c. The largest proportionate increase is projected to occur in the over-80-year age group
   d. The Hispanic and Asian population have the greatest variation in country of origin

3. To assist in assessing an elderly patient for manifestations of depression, which of the following tools would be most helpful?
   a. Mini Mental Status Exam
   b. Instrumental activities of daily living
   c. Geriatric depression scale
   d. Activities of daily living
4. When assessing a patient to confirm that he is experiencing pseudo dementia and not dementia, the nurse would identify which of the following as characteristic of pseudo dementia?
   a. Insidious onset of symptoms
   b. Answers typically with "I don't know"
   c. Fluctuations in mood and behavior
   d. Difficulties concealed by the patient
5. A nurse is instructing a patient in behavioral therapy techniques. These might include:
   a. Early conflict identification
   b. Modification of relationships
   c. Relaxation exercises
   d. Life review
6. The primary focus of care for an elderly patient with anxiety disorder is to:
   a. Encourage adaptation of more realistic thinking patterns
   b. Promote assertive behavior
   c. Improve communication
   d. Confront and overcome stress
7. When caring for the elderly patient with schizophrenia, the nurse would anticipate the use which of the following?
   a. ECT
   b. Psychodrama
   c. Music therapy
   d. Reminiscence therapy
8. When administering psychopharmacologic agents to elderly patients, the nurse is aware that the patient is at an increased risk for toxicity primarily because of changes in the drug's:
   a. Absorption
   b. Distribution
   c. Metabolism
   d. Excretion

Critical thinking exercises

1. Using the patient scenario in Nursing Care Plan 27-1 (in the textbook), Mr. V., and the chart below, identify possible biopsychosocial etiologies for this patient and develop appropriate biopsychosocial outcomes and interventions.

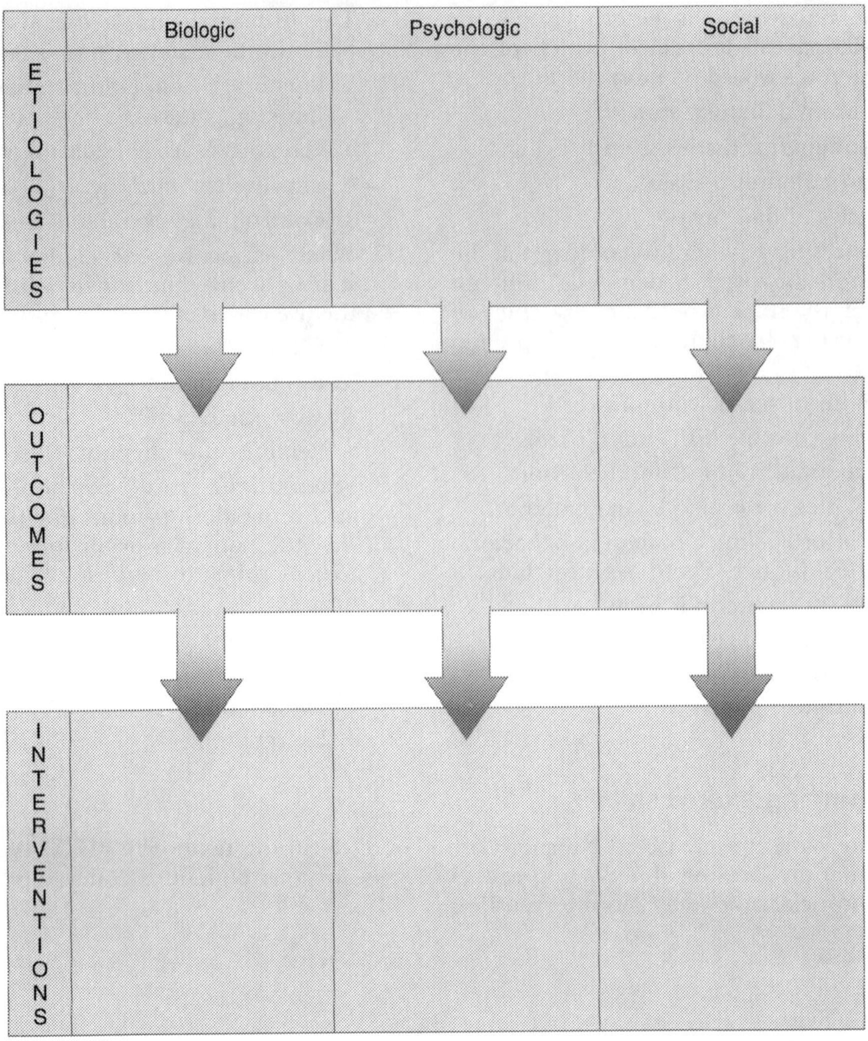

2. An 85-year-old German born male is admitted to a respite care facility for a two month stay, while his primary caretakers are away. His only child, a son, lives approximately 1500 miles away. On admission, the patient is alert and oriented ×3, joking and laughing, and telling stories about the past. His history reveals bilateral cataracts, heart failure, and degenerative joint disease. He is extremely hard of hearing, wearing a hearing aid in the left ear at all times. After approximately two weeks, the patient becomes extremely agitated, yelling and screaming at the staff. The chart reveals increased periods of confusion. "Nobody does anything right. Everybody's stealing my money."
   a. Evaluate this patient for normal age-related changes.

   b. Compare his behavior on admission with his behavior two weeks later. What might account for these changes?

   c. Develop an appropriate plan of care that addresses the patient's current needs.

3. An elderly patient, diagnosed with depression, is to receive venlafaxin hydrochloride. After researching this drug, prepare a teaching plan for the patient and his family addressing specific concerns for the elderly patient.

4. Visit an assisted living facility in your area. Evaluate the services provided and the populations served. How does this facility meet the needs of its residents?

5. Interview the family of a patient in residential care. Explore how the family came to their decision for this type of care.

28 ▪ *Care of the homeless mentally ill*

CHAPTER HIGHLIGHTS

Chapter 28 explores the care of the homeless mentally ill patient. It examines the possible risk factors for and the physical and psychological impact of homelessness along with the homeless person's access to health care. Using the nursing process framework, this chapter also addresses nursing management and possible community resources.

Chapter 28 key points include the following:

- Homeless persons, a heterogeneous group, include single men and women, single women with children, immigrants, those with severe and persistent mental illnesses and drug abuse, and those released from prison.
- Homelessness (not a choice) results from exhaustion of support systems, loss of income source or housing, flight from an abusive situation, or relapse into substance abuse.
- Although a comprehensive holistic nursing assessment is important, analysis of the mental status examination may prove the most critical data for planning care.
- An interdisciplinary approach capable of addressing the multiple needs of the homeless mentally ill patient and coordinating care delivery is most effective.
- Nurses need to confront stereotypes about the homeless and the mentally ill and view the patient as an individual with strengths and weaknesses.

STUDENT ACTIVITIES

Word unscramble

Below is a list of scrambled words. Unscramble each word and place it in the appropriate space next to its definition.

fienrctogiainit   laud sginoiads

hrnccoi fsadifnoiiatli   ssensselemoh

ilaestoazidintunitniot

______________ 1. The release of persons with severe and persistence mental illnesses from state mental hospitals to the community.

______________ 2. Lack of love and support from a solid network of family and friends.

______________ 3. Refurbishment of buildings and homes in run-down neighborhoods with subsequent increases in rent.

______________ 4. Presence of a psychoactive substance abuse and mental illness.

______________ 5. Living in a shelter, on the street, or other temporary living quarters for a sustained period of time.

Short answer

Write your answer to the question in the space provided.

1. Explain how deinstitutionalization has impacted the number of homeless individuals.

2. List the six principal risk factors for homelessness.

3. Identify the four categories of health problems associated with the homeless.

4. Name four common respiratory health problems seen in the homeless population.

5. State the most urgent need for the homeless person.

6. List six possible barriers that a homeless person must overcome for access to health care.

Self-exploration

1. On a sheet of paper, write down the characteristics that you believe to be applicable to the homeless. Examine this list for any stereotypical or judgmental items.

2. Imagine if you were homeless and living on the street.
   a. How would you satisfy your basic needs for shelter, nutrition, hygiene, and sleep?

   b. How would you maintain your safety?

   c. What would you do if you should become sick?

Multiple choice

Circle the option that best answers the question.

1. A patient comes to the clinic for evaluation. He is cleanly dressed and carrying a small satchel. The patient refuses to talk with the nurse about insurance coverage and is unwilling to provide an address. Closer examination leads the nurse to suspect that the patient may be homeless. Which of the following would be most helpful in eliciting more information about the patient's status?
   a. "You must tell me where you live."
   b. "You're homeless, aren't you?"
   c. "Tell me what your day is like."
   d. "Let's talk about where you sleep at night."

2. When planning care for a homeless person, the nurse needs to establish initial goals that:
   a. Meet all of the patient's needs
   b. Focus on the patient's basic needs
   c. Ensure a sense of belonging
   d. Address the patient's weaknesses

3. While speaking to a local community organization about the problem of homelessness, the nurse attempts to dispel some of the typical myths. Which of the following statements would help to dispel some of these myths?
   a. Most homeless persons suffer from mental illness
   b. Persons make a premeditated choice to be homeless
   c. All homeless persons abuse alcohol
   d. Homeless persons are more likely to be victims of crimes
4. When caring for a homeless patient, which of the following actions should be avoided?
   a. Making promises
   b. Identifying strengths
   c. Communicating with others
   d. Following through with statements
5. When assessing a homeless patient, the nurse needs to be aware of possible problems that are exacerbated by the exposure to the environment. Which of the following is an example of such a problem?
   a. Human immunodeficiency virus
   b. Scabies
   c. Peripheral vascular disease
   d. Seizures
6. Which of the following has been suggested as being the most vulnerable and most difficult group among the homeless to treat?
   a. Mentally ill homeless
   b. Substance abusing homeless
   c. Chronic physically ill homeless
   d. Dual diagnosis homeless
7. Prior to discharge, the person who typically assumes the responsibility of establishing the initial contact with the intended community service providers is the:
   a. Patient
   b. Nurse
   c. Physician
   d. Community service provider

Critical thinking exercises

1. For the activity listed in self-exploration exercise #1, compare your list with those of your fellow classmates. How are they similar? Different?

2. A patient with a dual diagnosis of substance abuse and schizophrenia is being discharged from the hospital following treatment for traumatic injuries sustained from a mugging. Using the discharge planning needs addressed in table 28-4 (in the textbook) and the elements in a comprehensive system of health care listed in table 28-3 (in the textbook), develop a plan of care for the patient after discharge.

29 ▪ *Special care concerns for persons with dual diagnosis*

CHAPTER HIGHLIGHTS

Chapter 29 examines the concept of dual diagnosis, the coexistence of a substance abuse disorder, and a mental health disorder. This chapter highlights assessment methods and explores the psychodynamics of their development. It also discusses specific mental illnesses and the adverse effects of concurrent substance abuse, providing possible treatment strategies and nursing interventions for the patient with a dual diagnosis.

Chapter 29 key points include the following:

- The incidence of substance abuse and one or more comorbid mental health disorders is very high.
- A dual diagnosis can consist of a primary mental illness and subsequent substance abuse, a primary substance abuse disorder and psychopathologic sequelae, dual primary diagnoses, or two disorders resulting from a common cause.
- Relapse is common in patients with dual diagnosis if both substance abuse disease and mental health disorder are not addressed concurrently.
- Barriers to effective treatment of dual diagnosis include: nature of substance abuse, countertransference and the position of substance abusers in society, misunderstandings about and stigmatization of mental illness, and underlying health issues.
- Alcohol and drug use can cause numerous mental health problems. These substances interact with common prescription and over-the-counter drugs to cause adverse reactions.
- Alcohol and drugs often exacerbate existing mental health disorders, possibly leading to noncompliance with prescribed medication regimen and other aspects of treatment.
- Treatment for patients with dual diagnosis include possible hospitalization, crisis stabilization, long-term treatment, medication management, patient education, use of self-help groups, relapse prevention, continuation of care, case management, and family support.
- Relapse prevention, crucial in treating dual diagnosis, includes analysis of high-risk situations for relapse, examination of cognitive, emotional, and behavioral components of high-risk situations, use of effective coping strategies, and available environmental supports.

STUDENT ACTIVITIES

Short answer

Write your answer to the question in the space provided.

1. When does the relapse cycle occur?

2. How did the community mental health reform movement affect the problem of dual diagnosis?

3. What are the four possible manifestations of a dual diagnosis?

4. How does the psychodynamic model view substance abuse?

5. Where are dually diagnosed patients more likely to be seen for primary health care?

6. What is the rationale for the importance of obtaining objective information for the dually diagnosed patient?

7. Why are benzodiazepines rarely used to treat patients with dual diagnosis of substance abuse and anxiety disorders?

8. ADHD is correlated with a high risk for what disorder?

9. What are the two main challenges to engaging dual diagnosis patients in treatment?

10. What are the principles of relapse prevention according to the Cenaps model?

Multiple choice

Circle the option that best answers the question.

1. When participating in a program designed to treat dual diagnosis, the nurse understands that which of the following is critical?
   a. Accessing crisis intervention
   b. Learning coping skills
   c. Establishing a positive social network
   d. Maintaining medication compliance
2. A patient diagnosed with post traumatic stress disorder began using cocaine to alleviate his anxiety symptoms. The nurse interprets this as which of the following manifestations of a dual diagnosis?
   a. A common etiology
   b. Dual primary diagnosis
   c. Primary substance abuse disorder with psychopathologic sequelae
   d. Primary mental illness with subsequent substance abuse
3. When discussing the possible barriers to obtain proper treatment for a patient with dual diagnosis, the nurse understands that which of the following is not considered a barrier?
   a. Patients attribute disturbing emotions to substance abuse
   b. Patients use the substance for the cure and not the cause of the distress
   c. Patients report substance abuse while seeking treatment for consequences
   d. Patients seek medications to alleviate symptoms caused by the abuse
4. When assessing the patient with a suspected dual diagnosis, it is most important for the nurse to do which of the following?
   a. Prioritize care based on how each diagnosis contributes to the severity of the current situation
   b. Rely on the patient's verbal and nonverbal reports of the problem
   c. Determine the primary disorder and plan appropriate interventions
   d. Anticipate the increased incidence of psychotic symptoms that will be present
5. When caring for the patient dually diagnosed with schizophrenia and substance abuse, nursing interventions typically include which of the following?
   a. Confront the patient's psychotic symptoms
   b. Help the patient identify areas of unmanageability
   c. Enlist the aid of the concept of a "higher power"
   d. Avoid referring to substance abuse as a disease

6. As part of treatment for a dually diagnosed patient with substance abuse and anxiety disorder, the patient is gradually exposed to the stressor and then progressively to more stressful stimuli triggers. The nurse correctly identifies this as which of the following?
   a. Environment restriction
   b. Positive self-talk
   c. Flooding
   d. Desensitization

7. A patient with bipolar disorder and substance abuse is being considered for chemical dependency treatment. Key to this patient's inclusion in the program is the patient's ability to do which of the following?
   a. Understand complex exercises
   b. Follow simple ground rules
   c. Correlate the disorders with behavior
   d. Refuse medications as appropriate

Critical thinking exercises

1. From the items listed in text box 29-2 (in the textbook), pick two topics and develop a teaching plan for an education group for patients with dual diagnosis.

2. Consider the following scenario. John M. is a 38-year-old divorced single, white man, who has received the dual diagnoses of alcohol dependency and bipolar disorder. He is currently unemployed and living with a friend. After drinking heavily for two days with his friend, Mr. M. borrowed the friend's car to go to the liquor store. He was stopped en route for erratic driving and cited for driving under the influence of alcohol. His speech was rambling, and he was unsteady on his feet. He asked to be taken to the local detoxification unit because "things were getting worse." There the counselors talked with him about sobriety and how to stay "clean." He never mentioned his bipolar disorder. After his detoxification, Mr. M. returned home and continued drinking.

   One week after discharge from the detoxification center, Mr. M was found near his friend's apartment. His speech was rambling, he acted suspicious, and he had threatened a neighbor, stating the he "had Mafia connections and that they would get him." County police took him to the psychiatric emergency department of a local community hospital, where he was admitted to the inpatient psychiatric unit on an involuntary, 72-hour hold as a danger to others. Within several hours, Mr. M. had calmed down and became tearful, explaining that he had stopped taking his medications recently because he had "felt great." When the 72-hour hold expired, he agreed to remain in the hospital and was stabilized on lithium carbonate. During his hospital stay, the issues of alcohol use and its relationship to his bipolar disorder were raised. He consented to entering the inpatient dual diagnosis program at the hospital to receive treatment for his psychiatric and substance abuse disorders.

   a. Analyze this scenario to determine the patient's priority needs.

   b. Develop an appropriate plan of care that addresses these priority needs.

30 ▪ Psychosocial aspects of medically compromised persons

CHAPTER HIGHLIGHTS

Chapter 30 examines the interplay of psychologic illness and physiologic disorders, including the medically ill person's risk for secondary mental illness. It explores the psychological impact of pain, possible psychopathologic complications of AIDs, and psychological illness related to trauma, CNS disorders, and acute and chronic medical illness, including possible biopsychosocial treatment interventions for each of these areas.

Chapter 30 key points include the following:

- Psychiatric illnesses are more common in persons with systemic or chronic medical illnesses than in others.
- Comorbid depression is commonly associated with endocrine and metabolic disturbances, viral infections, inflammatory disorders, and cardiopulmonary diseases.
- Anxiety disorders are commonly associated with Parkinson's disease, focal seizures, primary biliary cirrhosis, and chronic pain.
- Psychiatric illness accompanying medical illness is seldom recognized and treated. This is because psychiatric symptoms may precede the onset of disease symptoms, making it difficult to distinguish between the symptoms of the two conditions.
- The biologic basis of mental illness associated with medical illness is similar to that for the primary psychiatric illness. Thus similar biopsychosocial treatment strategies are effective.
- When mental illness occurs in medically ill persons, normal affective cognitive function critical to recovery and compliance with the medical treatment plan is affected. Therefore, presence of both conditions is potentially lethal.
- Mental health needs to be included in the standard health assessment of all medically ill persons and appropriate referrals need to be made.

STUDENT ACTIVITIES

Word find

Hidden within the following letter grid are key terms from chapter 30, listed below. The terms may be vertical, horizontal, diagonal, or backward. Circle the words as you find them.

Allodynia	Ischemia
Comorbidity	Kindling
Endorphin	Nociception
Hyperalgia	Serotonin


```
N I N O T O R E S P A C E
K N O C I C E P T I O N N
H I N O C O C E M P T I D
Y T N M S E R E P Y I H O
P H E O S K H I A F N P M
E C V R D C I X I S A R O
R S U B S T A N C E P O R
A O I I G O L S D T I D B
L M H D C A A I T L C N I
G P X I D L T N N R I E D
I L E T P L B E O G T N I
A I N Y D O L L A M Y I G
```

Fill in the blanks

Read each statement carefully and place the correct answer in the space(s) provided.

1. The balancing of essential levels of neurotransmitters is maintained by ________________.
2. The most common nociceptive transmitter released and transported along pain synapses in the presence of noxious stimuli is ________________.
3. The release of endorphins is mediated by ________________.
4. When events are interpreted as threatening, the ____________ initiates the stress response.
5. ____________ refers to the spontaneous recurrence of depressive illness associated with loss or trauma at an earlier age.
6. Hypoxia initiates the ________________.
7. Following a stroke, there is a generalized loss of ____________ activity and decreasing functional ability contributing to a depressed mood.
8. Physiologic evidence that pain perception involves pathways in the dorsal horn of the spinal cord that relay noxious stimuli to the brain forms the basis for the ____________ model.
9. Central pain, the underlying mechanism for most chronic pain, leads to ________________, ____________, and ________________.
10. Initially, the most common signs and symptoms of AIDs dementia complex are changes in ____________ and ________________.

Completion

Various treatment approaches to pain are listed below. Place the letter of the approach in the correct column on the chart.

a. Trigger point injection
b. Ibuprofen
c. Codeine
d. Amitryptyline
e. Lidocaine gel
f. Naloxone infusion
g. Behavioral psychotherapy
h. Clonidine
i. Phenytoin

First step	*Second step*	*Third step*	*Fourth step*

Multiple choice

Circle the option that best answers the question.

1. After evaluating assessment findings, the nurse determines that the patient is experiencing referred pain. The nurse understands that the biologic basis for this type of pain is the result of which of the following?
   a. Hyperalgia
   b. Plasticity
   c. Allodynia
   d. Hyperesthesia
2. When preparing to discuss the pain management program developed for a patient, which of the following statements by the patient would alert the nurse to the possibility that the program might not work?
   a. "I'm not sure my insurance will pay for these medicines."
   b. "I'll try to eat a salad every day to avoid constipation."
   c. "I'll call the doctor if my pain doesn't get better."
   d. "I know that I might need to try other medicines."
3. A review of a patient's history, admitted with manifestations of depression, reveals no recent significant stressors as a possible precipitating factor. The patient does report that at age 5, he witnessed both of his parents being shot and killed by an intruder. The nurse interprets this information, suspecting which of the following?
   a. Dissociative identity disorder
   b. Somatization disorder
   c. Kindling
   d. Agnosia
4. When dealing with the family of a patient who has suffered a stroke, the nurse is explaining about possible psychological complications. Which of the following would the nurse identify as the primary psychological disorder following a stroke?
   a. Dysfunctional grieving
   b. Panic disorder
   c. Obsessive-compulsive disorder
   d. Depression disorder
5. The nurse is attempting to identify whether a patient's signs and symptoms are the result of depression or his medical condition. Which of the following would be most likely related to his medical condition?
   a. Sleep disturbances
   b. Guilt feelings
   c. Low self-esteem
   d. Dissatisfaction with life
6. Which of the following drugs would the nurse anticipate administering to a patient with depression who is also medically ill?
   a. Monoamine oxidase inhibitors (MAOIs)
   b. Tricyclic antidepressants
   c. Benzodiazepines
   d. Serotonin selective reuptake inhibitors (SSRIs)
7. Which of the following statements by the nurse indicates a clear understanding of the interplay between medical and mental illness.
   a. "The treatment for the medical condition will not interfere with the treatment for the mental illness."
   b. "Drug therapy is the treatment of choice for both mental and physical disorders."
   c. "Chronic physical illness is a stressor that can increase psychological distress and risk for mental illness."
   d. "Measures are available to help prevent the occurrence of medical and mental illnesses."
8. An elderly patient with Parkinson's disease is receiving Amantidine. The patient begins to experience mental status changes including confusion, irritability, depression, and hallucinations. The nurse should anticipate the need for which of the following?
   a. Increasing the dosage of Amantidine by one-half the current dose
   b. Withholding the next dose, pending laboratory results
   c. Decreasing the dosage by one-half the current dose
   d. Administering the next dose with another prescribed agent

Critical thinking exercises

1. In your clinical area, review the charts of several patients who are experiencing pain. After checking with your clinical instructor, interview one of these patients and assess the patient's level of pain using the pain assessment tool listed in text box 30-3 (in the textbook). Present your findings to your clinical group for discussion, addressing the impact of the patient's pain on his physical and mental health.

2. Imagine the following clinical scenario. Mrs. M. V. is a widowed 52-year-old communications department manager who experienced a left hemisphere cerebrovascular accident (CVA) that resulted in right hemiparesis. Mrs. V has successfully completed rehabilitation, wears a leg brace to correct right footdrop, and is able to ambulate with a four-point walker. She was able to return to work but recently has begun to find it difficult to go to work. Mrs. V has always experienced periods of "low energy" and relates that her mother had periods of "down moods" that caused her to stay in bed for weeks at a time. After her stroke and rehabilitation, Mrs. V. began to experience various somatic complaints and to feel "sad" and hopeless as she realized rehabilitation would not restore function to her right extremities. She reports sleeplessness, fatigue, and anorexia. She was admitted with reports of severe headache, increased hemiparesis, weight loss of 30 pounds and visual abnormalities. She has stopped smoking at the time of her CVA, denies alcohol and caffeine use, and takes her antihypertensive medication and insulin. She is single and currently lives alone. Her past medical history is positive for insulin dependent diabetes for 5 years using regular insulin, 5 units each morning, and lente insulin, 5 units every evening, hypertension controlled with hydrochlorothiazide, 35 mg b.i.d., and a history of cataracts. She has no known drug allergies.

   Physical examination: Thin, well-dressed, alert, oriented white female with no dysarthria.

   Cardiopulmonary exam: Normal. Blood pressure in both arms 140/86 and pulse 82.

   Neurologic exam: Extremity strength 4/5 on right; 5/5 on left. Sensation decreased to pinprick in right and left lower extremities over the foot up to mid calf.

   Laboratory results: Hematology, thyroid function, liver and renal function tests within normal limits; blood sugar 120 mg/dL.

   A diagnosis of secondary depression related to CVA was made.

   Develop a plan of care that addresses this patient's priority needs.

3. You are assigned to care for the following patient. Mr. B. K, a 30-year-old dental hygiene clinic employee has been evaluated in another clinic for multiple episodes of dizziness, palpitations, severe headaches, feelings of suffocation, and difficulty swallowing and catching his breath. These symptoms have been relatively minor for about one year but became more frightening in the past 3 months. He complained of feelings of being smothered, severe apprehension, increased palpitations, insomnia, and constant restlessness. He reported chronic fatigue and constant head and neck aches.

   His past medical history is negative for chest pain, syncope, and medical illness, but positive for hay fever. The history revealed untreated hypertension. He reports social drinking (0 to 2 glasses of wine per week), smoking one-half pack of cigarettes per day, drinking several cups of regular coffee daily, and inactivity. He has no known drug allergies.

   For several years, his medications have included triprolidine (Actifed) prn for hay fever (6 to 10 tablets weekly) and albuterol (Proventil), two puffs t.i.d. as needed for allergies to tree pollen, grasses, and cat fur. He admitted to taking more than two puffs on many occasions, to overcome the feeling of suffocation.

   He is single and lives with a same-sex partner. HIV infection was recently diagnosed in his significant other. Family history is negative for mental illness, stroke, thyroid disease, and diabetes.

   Physical examination: Well-nourished, well-developed, cooperative white male appearing his stated age.

   Vital signs: Blood pressure 170/90 ×3, lying, sitting, and standing, taken 6 minutes apart; pulse 120 and regular.

   Cardiopulmonary exam: Within normal limits

   Neurologic exam: Mild hemiparesis of distal right hand 4/5

   Remainder of physical exam: Unremarkable

Laboratory tests: Chest X ray, CBC, hemoglobin and hematocrit within normal limits; thyroxine normal; fasting cholesterol 214 mg/dL; HIV negative; head CT normal

A diagnosis of generalized anxiety disorder was made.

Using the information from this situation, identify possible biopsychosocial etiologies for this patient and develop appropriate biopsychosocial outcomes and interventions.

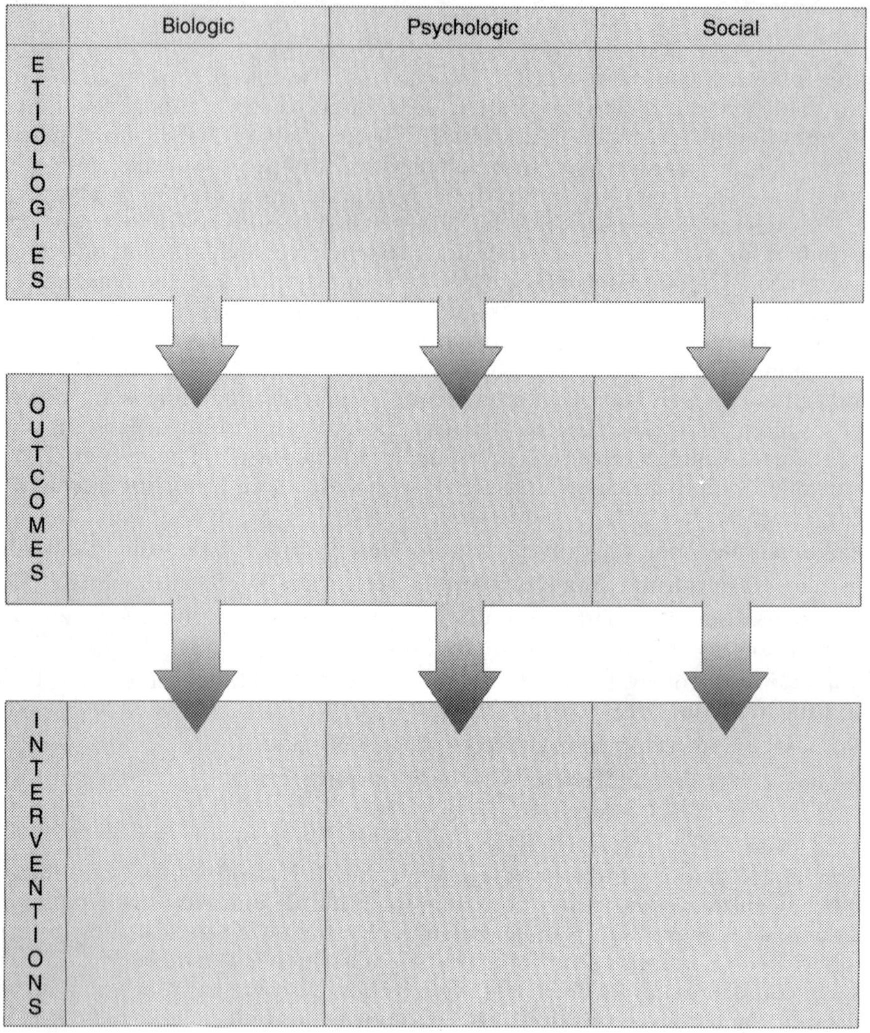

4. As part of a class exercise, you are asked to walk around your environment and carry out your usual activities wearing a stone in one of your shoes to simulate the experience of pain. This simulation is to last for approximately one hour.
   a. How did this experience of pain impact your activities?

   b. What feelings were evoked while you were in pain?

   c. What coping strategies did you use?

   d. Did the knowledge that the pain would soon be relieved influence your reactions? If so, how?

   e. Imagine if this pain was chronic. Would you react or feel differently? Why or why not?

UNIT SIX
Care challenges in psychiatric nursing

31 ▪ *Biopsychosocial aspects of stress and crisis*

CHAPTER HIGHLIGHTS

Chapter 31 addresses the inevitability of stress and crisis on all individuals. It examines the antecedents to stress addressing the person-environment relationship, physiologic and emotional responses to stress, coping, and adaptation. This chapter explores crisis and identifies the types of crises including the crisis event, such as death of a loved one. Using a nursing process approach and biopyschosocial framework, this chapter describes the nursing management for the patient experiencing stress or crisis.

Chapter 31 key points include the following:

- When the person-environment relationship is appraised as unfavorable, stress occurs.
- Simultaneous emotional and physiologic stress responses lead to an innate tendency to act.
- Personal factors such as personality patterns, beliefs, values, and commitment to an outcome interact with environmental demands and constraints that produce a person-environment relationship.
- Social support, within a social network, can help a person cope with stress.
- Problem-focused or emotion-focused coping can be effective. When successful, enhanced health, psychological well-being, and social functioning are enhanced.
- A crisis is a severely stressful situation causing an exaggerated stress response. The nursing process, similar to that for the person experiencing a stress response, focuses on increased attention to safety issues.

STUDENT ACTIVITIES

Matching

Place the letter of description from the righthand column next to the correct term in the lefthand column.

_______ 1. Cognitive appraisal
_______ 2. Coping
_______ 3. Social network
_______ 4. Problem focused coping
_______ 5. Constraints
_______ 6. Adaptation
_______ 7. Social support
_______ 8. Crisis
_______ 9. Emotion focused coping
_______ 10. Social functioning

a. Harmonious interpersonal interactions
b. Personal and environmental limitations
c. Change in the meaning of the situation through reinterpretation without a change in the person-environment relationship
d. Capacity to survive and flourish
e. Performance of daily activities within the context of interpersonal relations and family and community roles
f. Examination of the environment for negotiation with personal goals and beliefs
g. Attack on the source of stress through elimination
h. Management of demands and emotions generated by appraisal
i. Defined set of persons involving personal contacts
j. Severely stressful situation with failure of coping mechanisms and lack of adaptation

True/false

Determine whether each sentence below is true or false. If true, write true in the space below. If false, rewrite the sentence to be true.

_______ 1. Being under stress is usually viewed as a positive experience because the outcomes are positive.
_______ 2. The person and environment are two important antecedents to the stress response.
_______ 3. Two important concepts related to social networks include intensity and reciprocity.
_______ 4. Social dissupport, relationships that hinder growth, are emotionally destructive and deplete resources.
_______ 5. Health is positively affected when coping is effective.
_______ 6. Stress responses are similar from one person to another.
_______ 7. Acting impulsively implies few real coping skills.
_______ 8. Minimizing the seriousness of a problem is an example of problem-focused coping.
_______ 9. A crisis can typically last for an indefinite period of time.
_______ 10. Bereavement usually follows resolution of a crisis.
_______ 11. With dysfunctional grieving, the bereaved becomes a chronic mourner fixed on the deceased and events surrounding the death.
_______ 12. In a crisis, the person's social network is often disrupted.

Self-exploration

1. Using the Recent Life Changes questionnaire found in table 31-2 (in the textbook), evaluate yourself for life change events. Then analyze your score to determine your risk for illness.

2. Look back on a time when you felt stressed.
   a. How did you respond physically?

b. How did you respond emotionally?

c. Identify your emotions using the categories cited by Lazarus.

d. Did you use problem-focused or emotion-focused coping?

e. Compare your response and coping methods with your fellow classmates.

Multiple choice

Circle the option that best answers the question.

1. An instructor, explaining the various functions of social support, cites which of the following as an example of tangible support?
   a. Giving advice to another
   b. Confiding in someone
   c. Providing feedback
   d. Taking someone to the store
2. A daughter is caring for her terminally ill mother with the aid of a hospice organization. The hospice nurse identifies the nursing diagnosis of "caregiver role strain." Which of the following best supports this nursing diagnosis?
   a. Social network and support is limited because of the home environment
   b. Daughter is committed to having the mother die at home
   c. The patient's demands take priority over the caregiver's needs
   d. The daughter is demonstrating type A personality behaviors
3. A nurse is preparing a class about the effect of stress on the immune system for a local support group comprised of family members of patients with Alzheimer's disease. When preparing the presentation, the nurse understands which of the following?
   a. Negative moods promote immune activity
   b. Cortisol contributes to reduced lymphocyte numbers
   c. Increased norepinephrine levels enhance immune function
   d. Stress elevates white blood cell counts
4. Which of the following interventions would be appropriate for a generalist nurse to institute?
   a. Cognitive restructuring
   b. Touch therapy
   c. Guilt work
   d. Limit setting
5. A patient comes to the clinic complaining of anxiety and helplessness. Assessment reveals that he had experienced an apartment fire two weeks ago in which his roommate suffered extensive burns and smoke inhalation. He received only minor first degree burns on his arms and legs. Since that time, the patient reports recurrent dreams and flashbacks about the fire, so much so that he is finding it difficult to work. He states, "I feel like I'm in a fog all the time." Based on this assessment, the nurse interprets these findings as an indication of:
   a. Generalized anxiety disorder
   b. Developmental crisis disorder
   c. Acute stress disorder
   d. Somatoform disorder
6. The son of a patient who has recently died reports that he is angry and irritable, stating, "I've stopped calling my friends because I just can't talk about my parent's death." The nurse correctly identifies that the son is in which of the following stages of grief?
   a. Shock and disbelief
   b. Acute mourning: Intense feeling
   c. Acute mourning: Social withdrawal
   d. Resolution
7. In a crisis, referring a family to appropriate community resources helps to accomplish which of the following?
   a. Strengthening social networks to reduce effects of crisis
   b. Providing accurate information for problem solving
   c. Understanding the significance of the crisis
   d. Facing the reality to resolve the crisis

8. During a crisis, priority nursing interventions focus on which of the following needs?
   a. Safety
   b. Self-esteem
   c. Belonging
   d. Socialization
9. The physician orders lorazepam (Ativan), 0.5 mg t.i.d., for an elderly patient. The nurse would instruct the patient about which of the following?
   a. Stopping the drug immediately if the patient becomes lightheaded
   b. Dangling at the side of the bed before getting up out of bed
   c. Expecting to have some difficulty urinating
   d. Avoiding taking the drug with food
10. A patient is identified as exhibiting type B personality behaviors. The nurse would expect to find which of the following?
   a. Easily satisfied
   b. Impatience
   c. Restlessness
   d. Hostility

Critical thinking exercises

1. Imagine that you are the nurse in the following clinical scenario. Connie is the fifth of twelve children. She was reared in a small German-American community as a strict Roman Catholic. Her father, a local fireman, died from a heart attack when Connie was in college. By baby-sitting, her mother was able to support the children who still lived at home. Connie was able to complete college and then moved away from home to teach. She married a man who also taught school and was deeply religious. Connie never really enjoyed having sex with her husband, but she believed that it was her "wifely duty." After five years of marriage, Connie was seduced by another female teacher, who awakened Connie's sexuality. Connie quietly divorced her husband but never told her family of her sexual orientation. She felt guilty about her lesbian lifestyle, which violated the values of her strict religious upbringing. She stopped attending church.

   As Connie's mother grew older, her arthritis become worse and she was no longer able to babysit. By the time Connie's youngest sister was old enough to go to college, Connie's other brothers and sisters were married and had children, with the exception of one sister who had joined a religious order. Connie decided to return to her small community and live with her mother. She was hired by the local parochial high school as a science teacher. She is 38 years old.

   Connie's mother initially required little care. Connie developed her own social network and was frequently gone on weekends. As her mother became more disabled, Connie curtailed her own social life to care for her mother and assume more of the household responsibilities. She refused to ask her brothers and sisters to help care for their mother because they had their own lives. On the other hand, she became increasingly angry with them because "they don't understand or care about my burden." Gradually, within two years, Connie was spending every weekend at home cooking and cleaning for the approaching week. Her mother became more depressed and irritable. Connie found herself having arguments with her mother and began to regret having returned home. Connie also became irritable, resentful, and depressed. She spent most evenings watching television and eating. During a two-year period, she gained fifty pounds. She did not participate in any extracurricular activities at school or maintain contact with her friends. She had frequent crying spells and she missed her friends, her former lifestyle, and even her church.

   On Christmas day, Connie's mother was hospitalized for chest pain. The plan was that Connie's mother would return home once her condition had been stabilized. Her mother's primary nurse met with Connie for discharge planning. The nurse noticed that Connie appeared tense and looked very tired. During the discharge planning, it became obvious to the nurse that Connie found her caregiving responsibilities stressful.

   Develop a plan of care that addresses Connie's priority needs. For each nursing diagnosis identified, list the defining characteristics and related factors.

2. The following nursing diagnoses (see p. 135) have been identified for a person experiencing stress. For each nursing diagnosis, identify the defining characteristics and propose appropriate outcomes.

Nursing diagnosis	*Defining characteristics*	*Possible outcomes*
Anxiety		
Coping, ineffective individual		
Decisional conflict		
Fear		
Social interaction, impaired		
Social isolation		

3. Using the clinical vignette, " Stress and Students," described in text box 31-2 (in the textbook), analyze each student's stress response incorporating the factors involved in the person-environment relationship and cognitive appraisal.

32 ▪ *Biopsychosocial management of aggression and violence*

CHAPTER HIGHLIGHTS

Chapter 32 explores the concepts of aggression and violence. It examines the models of anger and aggression, and the relevance of these concepts to nursing. Applying the nursing process with integration of the biopsychosocial framework, this chapter describes the nursing management of the person experiencing anger, aggression, and violence.

Chapter 32 key points include the following:

- Three types of biopsychosocial theories are used to explain anger, aggression, and violence: neurobiologic (cognitive neuroassociation, neurostructural, and neurochemical models), psychological (psychoanalytic, behavioral, and cognitive theories), and sociologic (sociocultural and interactional theories).
- The potential for expression of aggressive and violent behaviors is increased by internal and external influences. Internal influences include biologic, thought processing, or sensory impairment; external influences include interactional processes, beliefs held by the nurse, and workplace culture.
- Patient aggression and violence are serious concerns for nurses in all areas of clinical practice. Training in and policies and procedures for the prevention and management of aggressive episodes should be available.
- Intervention choices include biologic, affective, cognitive, behavioral, and environmental.

STUDENT ACTIVITIES

Word unscramble

Below is a list of scrambled words. Unscramble each word and place it in the appropriate space next to its definition.

mioaenotl irctuic	sstieaervsens
ggarseiosn	iounabdres
rgena	

_____________ 1. Open, direct, honest, and confident behavior and communication.

_____________ 2. Negative emotion occurring when there is a threat, delay, or thwarting of a goal.

_____________ 3. Defining limits of persons, objects, or relationships.

_____________ 4. Physical act of force

_____________ 5. Interrelationship between the limbic system, frontal lobe, and other parts of the brain.

Labeling

Each of the following statements are associated with a theoretical explanation for anger, aggression, and violence. Place the corresponding letter in the appropriate circle on the biopsychosocial illustration.

a. Instinctual impulses and events in the environment that stimulate release of instinctual urge
b. Inequities in relationships with one person subordinate to a superior one
c. Emotional circuit to determine the meaning a person gives to a situation
d. Lower than average level of serotonin in cerebrospinal fluid
e. Rewards for expression of anger and violence
f. Using reason, with perceived threats based on distorted perceptions, lead to aggressive and violent behaviors
g. Response based on interpretation of an experience depending on prior experience and associations
h. Anger and violence as a response to interference with a goal
i. Expression of aggression positively correlated with a coercive style
j. Inappropriate negative emotions stemming from irrational beliefs

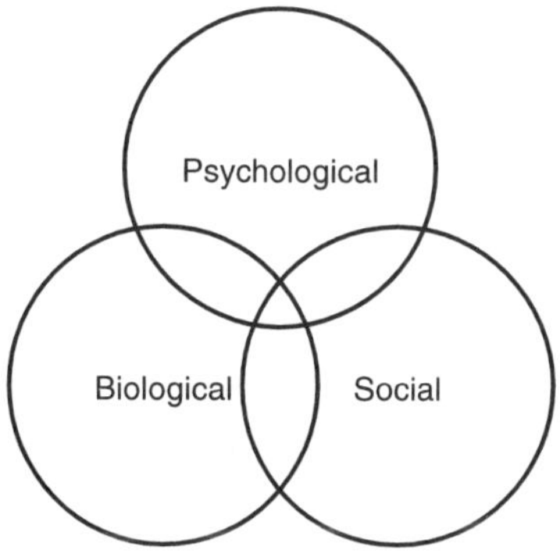

Multiple choice

Circle the option that best answers the question.

1. When assessing a patient for the potential for aggression and violence, the nurse identifies which of the following as crucial?
   a. History of central nervous system dysfunction
   b. Presence of disordered perceptions
   c. Missed doses of medications
   d. Sensory hearing loss
2. When viewing aggression and violence from a circular causality, the nurse typically does which of the following?
   a. Attempts to understand the link between behaviors
   b. Labels the patient as the problem and other factors as secondary
   c. Decides to gain control over the patient's behavior
   d. Determines who is to blame
3. When planning interventions for the patient with anger and aggression, it is important that the nurse remember which of the following?
   a. All patients have a right to express anger in any way they feel comfortable
   b. It is the nurse's responsibility to determine alternatives to violent outbursts
   c. Anger is a normal emotion expressed by all persons of any age and culture
   d. In most instances, the patient cannot assume responsibility for the behavior
4. When interacting with a patient in the day room, the nurse determines that a violent outburst is imminent. Which of the following actions should the nurse do first?
   a. Talk to the patient calmly
   b. Give the patient choices
   c. Remove the other patients
   d. Call for help

5. The physician orders paroxetine (Paxil) for a patient with a history of alcohol abuse who is aggressive and violent. When caring for this patient, the nurse would expect to monitor which of the following?
   a. Urinary output
   b. Liver function tests
   c. White blood cell count
   d. Serum glucose levels
6. A patient decides to remove herself from the day room because she is beginning to experience feelings of aggression. When talking with the patient later in the day, the nurse praises the patient's actions. The nurse is using which of the following techniques?
   a. Validation
   b. Exploration
   c. Commendation
   d. Thought stopping
7. Which of the following interventions would most likely increase rather than decrease the potential for violent behavior?
   a. Monitoring the items brought in by the family and other visitors
   b. Using paper plates and plastic utensils for meals
   c. Placing two potentially violent patients in the same room
   d. Having the patient use an electric razor for shaving

Critical thinking exercises

1. Compare and contrast assertiveness and aggression. Create a checklist of behaviors characteristic of each.

2. Imagine if you were assigned to care for a patient who experienced a spinal cord injury resulting in paralysis from his waist down. After physical therapy one day, upon entering his room, the patient screams, "Get out of here. I don't want to see anyone, especially you." He picks up a plant sitting on his overbed table and throws it at you, just barely missing you.
   a. How would you respond in this situation?

   b. What feelings might you experience?

   c. Would these feelings interfere with your ability to care for this patient? Please explain why or why not.

3. Consider this scenario. Mr. B. is a 26-year-old newly divorced man admitted to an inpatient psychiatric unit of a general hospital following an overdose two days ago, after his divorce was finalized. He was extremely distraught because of losing the custody of his only child and being mandated to pay what, in his opinion, was excessive child support. He has been treated for bipolar I disorder for several years. His only other depressive episode occurred four years ago after the death of both parents in a tragic accident. After a stormy marriage, his wife of six years left him, taking their 3-year-old son with her. Mr. B has one brother whom he rarely sees. He is employed as an electrician and makes a good income. Currently his medications include Lithium carbonate, 300 mg b.i.d., Prozac, 20 mg daily, and Haldol, 4 mg prn, for agitation.

   Since his admission, Mr. B. has been cooperative but has not provided many details about his personal life. He admits that the arguments with his ex-wife occasionally became "physical." When discussing his divorce, he becomes very agitated. However, the rest of his time is spent quietly in his room or in the hall. He is restless when in the company of other patients. On the third day of hospitalization, Mr. B. becomes very edgy. His tone of voice is angry and he begins pacing. When approached by another patient, he is verbally abusive.
   a. Analyze this situation for possible biopsychosocial etiologies.

   b. Develop an appropriate plan of care addressing Mr. B.'s priority needs, including his verbally abusive behavior.

33 ▪ Biopsychosocial aspects of caring for abused persons

CHAPTER HIGHLIGHTS

Chapter 33 reviews the care of persons, specifically children, elders, and women, who are the victims and survivors of abuse. It explores the possible theories used to explain abuse and describes the types of abuse and its victims. Using a nursing process approach and biopsychosocial framework, this chapter explores the nursing management for each type of abuse.

Chapter 33 key points include the following:

- Nurses need to be aware of the abuse of children, women, and elders as a national health problem.
- Many theories have been attempted to explain abuse.
- A cycle of violence consisting of three phases of increasing frequency and severity is well documented.
- Child abuse, whether physical, sexual, neglectful, or emotional leaves many scars that can result in problems in adulthood.
- Elder abuse may be physical, emotional, neglectful, or financial.
- Responses to abuse may include depression, acute stress disorder, post traumatic stress syndrome, and dissociative identity disorder.
- Knowledge of the signs and symptoms of abuse and vigilant assessment are important for all nurses.
- Nurses can help victims of abuse to view themselves as survivors.

STUDENT ACTIVITIES

Matching

Place the letter of the statement from the righthand column next to the theory it correctly describes in the lefthand column.

_______ 1. Psychoanalytic theories
_______ 2. Social learning theories
_______ 3. Feminist theories
_______ 4. Neurobiologic theories
_______ 5. Sociologic theories

a. Patriarchal society perpetuating the attitudes to support violence
b. Decreased levels of 5-HIAA influences impulsive behavior and violence
c. Lack of impulse control
d. Cultural norms permit violent behavior
e. Intergenerational transmission of violence

Short answer

Write your answer to the question in the space provided.

1. Name three characteristics of a patriarchal society that are believed to perpetuate violence against women.

2. List three factors that suggest the relationship of alcohol to violence.

3. State the single greatest cause of serious injury to women.

4. Identify the two common structural components found in most abusive relationships.

5. Name the three major childhood rights violated by all forms of child abuse.

6. Describe the difference in behavior of abused boys and girls.

7. Identify six characteristics that place an elderly person at greater risk for abuse.

8. State the most common biologic response to abuse.

9. List three typical psychological responses commonly seen with survivors of abuse.

10. Name the theory that explains why the cycle of violence is so powerful in entrapping women in a violent relationship.

Self-exploration

1. You are assigned to role-play the following situation. An elderly female patient with a history of multiple health problems currently living with his son and daughter-in-law is admitted to the facility with soft tissue injuries and fractures to the left humerus and wrist. This patient has been seen in the emergency department numerous times over the last year with similar types of injuries. Elder abuse is suspected. You are the nurse assigned to care for this patient.
   a. How would you feel in this situation? Be sure to identify your feelings, beliefs, and values about elder abuse.

   b. Would any of these you just identified interfere with your caring for this patient? If yes, explain how. If no, explain why.

   c. What measures could you take to ensure that you provide the optimal care for this patient and his family?

2. Imagine that you were caring for a patient who, during a conversation, reveals to you that he occasionally "hits his wife."
   a. How would you react to this statement and the patient?

   b. Would your reaction be different if the patient was the recipient rather than the inflictor? Please explain.

Multiple choice

Circle the option that best answers the question.

1. When explaining to a group of battered women about the connection between alcohol and violence, the nurse is correct in stating that alcohol:
   a. Is the primary cause of violent acts
   b. Is one of many contributing factors
   c. Is more closely associated with emotional abuse
   d. Plays no role in sexual abuse
2. While assessing a woman who is in an abusive relationship, the nurse would expect which of the following?
   a. Feelings of dependency
   b. Feeling of omnipotence
   c. Consistent aversive conditions
   d. Weak affective bond with partner
3. Two children, a 5-year-old and a 2-year-old, are burned in a house fire because the 5-year-old was left to watch the 2-year-old while the mother went down to the corner store to buy a pack of cigarettes. While away, the children were playing with matches left on the coffee table and a fire started. This is an example of which of the following?
   a. Emotional neglect
   b. Physical neglect
   c. Failure to protect
   d. Medical neglect
4. The nurse would anticipate finding which of the following behaviors when assessing a school-aged female child who has been abused?
   a. Overt aggressiveness
   b. Fights with schoolmates
   c. Temper tantrums
   d. Clinging to others
5. A patient with a history of sexual abuse as a child is diagnosed with a dissociative identity disorder. Assessment findings would include which of the following?
   a. External generalized voice hallucinations
   b. Forgetfulness about the traumatic events
   c. Two or more distinct personality states
   d. Ignorance of the reality of the hallucinations
6. When assessing a patient who is the victim of abuse, the most important step is:
   a. Reporting the incident of abuse
   b. Establishing a trusting nurse-patient relationship
   c. Evaluating the patient for physical injuries
   d. Evaluating the patient for substance abuse
7. When faced with a situation involving child abuse, the nurse's priority is to:
   a. Provide for the safety of the child
   b. Treat any health concerns and problems
   c. Break the secret of violence
   d. Teach the child how to trust
8. When reviewing class notes in preparation for an examination about the possible theories of abuse, the student identifies which of the following as an underlying belief of the psychoanalytic theory?
   a. Exposure to violence in the family promotes violent family members
   b. Violent behavior is accepted as normal by society
   c. Battering results from deficient coping skills
   d. Women are inherently inferior to men
9. A victim of child abuse may exhibit which of the following short-term consequences?
   a. Sexual maladjustment
   b. Psychosomatic symptoms
   c. Major depression
   d. Revictimization
10. A patient with post traumatic stress disorder has a history of drug dependency. Which of the following medications would the nurse know to be contraindicated?
    a. Tricyclic antidepressants
    b. Benzodiazepines
    c. SSRIs
    d. MAOIs

Critical thinking exercises

1. You are assigned to care for the following patient. Mrs. J is a 25-year-old married woman of Hispanic descent who visited the primary care facility for treatment of a dislocated shoulder. She is accompanied by her husband of 18 months, who insists on remaining with her. Over his protests and after being informed that it is agency policy that all examinations be conducted in private, Mrs. J enters the examination room. She appears frightened. During the assessment, Mrs. J relates that she fell down the stairs at home while carrying a basket of laundry. She has several bruises on her neck and face, some of which appear to be more recent than others. Her chart indicated that she has come on several occasions with various vague somatic complaints. On being questioned about her other injuries, Mrs. J. begins crying and says that her husband has been beating her and she is afraid that he might kill her someday.

   Mrs. J and her husband grew up in the same community and their parents attended the same church. Mrs. J, who worked as a bank teller, lived at home until she married. Encouraged by her family, she married Mr. J. (who was recently discharged from the Navy). Since Mr. J.'s job paid well, she quit her job at the bank to stay home. Since her marriage, Mrs. J's husband has become increasingly controlling of her activities, to the point that she cannot go outside the house; he calls her throughout the day to monitor her whereabouts. He checks the telephone bills to monitor her calls and checks the gas mileage on the car to make sure that she is telling the truth about her daily activities. He has not allowed her to see any friends for over six months. She is allowed to see her family only when he is present. If he has any reason to suspect that she has lied about her daily activities, "He slaps me around and shoves me into the wall." On one recent occasion, he beat her up for taking a shower while he was at work. He reasoned that if she needed a shower, that must mean that she had been unfaithful.

   While the couple were dating, Mr. J was possessive and did not like Mrs. J talking to other men. He also called her frequently during the day. However, she was flattered by the attention and did not think much about it. But things became progressively worse. At first, Mr. J. used violence only occasionally and seemed genuinely remorseful after each incident, promising that it would never happen again. Now, he has been hitting her almost weekly with increasing force. Mrs. J. relates that she tried to leave but that her husband got home before she could get away. She relates that he has hunting guns and knives in the house, and she believes that he is capable of using them.

   Mrs. J. reports that she is having difficulty sleeping because of vivid nightmares. She feels "jumpy and scared all the time." She reports feeling trapped and helpless to change her situation. She also reports that she has been using alcohol on a regular basis to "help me sleep and to calm me down."

   Develop an appropriate plan of care that addresses Mrs. J.'s priority needs. For each nursing diagnosis, list the defining characteristics and related factors.

2. Using the scenario in question #1, apply the cycle of violence, describing specific incidents from the scenario to support each phase of the cycle.

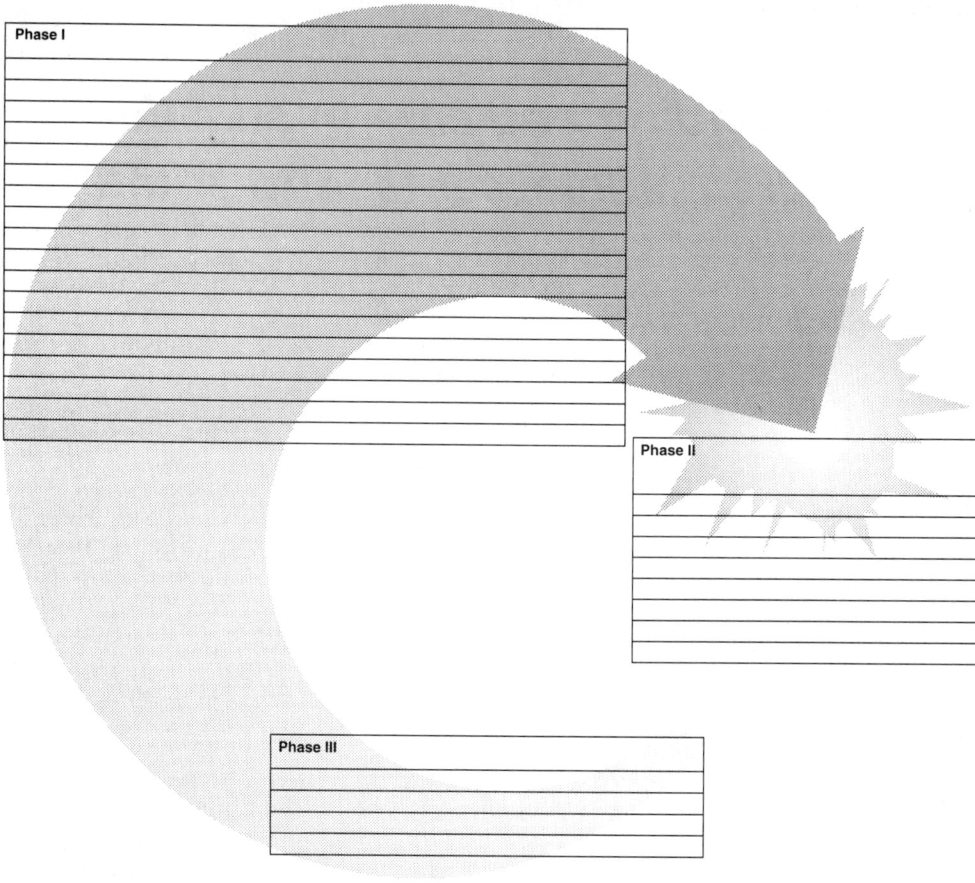

3. The following nursing diagnoses are listed on a plan of care for a patient who is a victim of violence. For each nursing diagnosis, identify the defining characteristics and propose appropriate outcomes.

Nursing diagnosis	*Defining characteristics*	*Possible outcomes*
Posttrauma response		
Powerlessness		
Social isolation		
Ineffective individual coping		
Self-esteem disturbance		
Ineffective family coping		

34 ▪ Case-finding and care in suicide: Children, adolescents, and adults

CHAPTER HIGHLIGHTS

Chapter 34 explores the concept of suicide, parasuicide, and suicidal ideation. It examines the epidemiology of suicidal behavior across the life span, etiology of suicide, and its impact on others. Applying the nursing process with integration of the biopsychosocial framework, this chapter describes the nursing management of the suicidal patient.

Chapter 34 key points include the following:

- Suicide is a common and major health problem occurring in 15 percent of all cases of major depression.
- Suicide completion is more common in males, specifically elderly males. Among women, it is most prevalent in white professional women.
- The increasing availability of firearms and alcohol corresponds to the rising rates of adolescent suicide.
- Parasuicide is more common among women than men.
- Persons attempting suicide most commonly do not seek medical or psychiatric assistance.
- Suicidal behavior is associated with family pedigree and has genetic and biologic origins.
- Persons threatening suicide have civil rights that must be maintained.
- The no-suicide contract is one means of increasing the suicidal patient's safety in the community.
- Voluntary hospitalization is the method of choice if hospitalization is necessary.
- The major objective of brief hospital care includes maintaining patient safety, reestablishing the patient's biologic equilibrium, strengthening the patient's coping skills, and developing an outpatient support system.
- The nurse caring for suicidal patients is vulnerable to secondary trauma and must take steps to maintain personal mental health.

STUDENT ACTIVITIES

Matching

Place the letter of the description from the righthand column next to the correct item in the lefthand column.

_______ 1. Suicide
_______ 2. Parasuicide
_______ 3. Suicidal ideation
_______ 4. Lethality
_______ 5. Competence
_______ 6. Case-finding

a. Thinking about and planning one's own death with doing self-harm
b. Degree of probability of successful completion of voluntarily taking one's own life
c. Sufficient judgment to legally enter into an agreement
d. Voluntarily killing one's self
e. Inquiry about the emotional symptoms a patient is having
f. Failed attempt to end one's life voluntarily

Short answer

Write your answer to the question in the space provided.

1. For each of the following statements about suicide, identify whether the theory is biologic, psychological, or social.
   a. Anger and aggression turned inward ______
   b. Downregulation of imidazoline receptor protein ______
   c. Distressed significant relationship ______
   d. Maladaptive coping mechanism ______
   e. Real or perceived loss of a significant object ______
2. List the three factors that can be used to determine lethality of suicide.
3. Identify the ages when suicide tends to be most prevalent.
4. Name the one factor that has been linked to thoughts about suicide in adulthood.
5. Describe the effect of suicide on grief.
6. Identify the nursing responsibilities for suicide prevention in the outpatient setting.
7. List four psychiatric diagnoses associated with suicide completion.
8. Describe the items needed for suicide to succeed.

Multiple choice

Circle the option that best answers the question.

1. When determining that involuntary hospitalization is required for a suicidal patient, the nurse must keep in mind that the only legal reason for such an action is that the patient:
   a. Cannot be safe in the community
   b. Is a danger to self or others
   c. Violates the no-suicide contract
   d. Is exhibiting increased suicidal ideation
2. When assessing a patient's risk for suicide, the nurse would expect which of the following patients to be at the greatest risk?
   a. Widowed elderly male living alone with a chronic illness
   b. An alcoholic female in recovery
   c. A middle-aged woman with depressive symptoms
   d. An adolescent whose uncle completed suicide
3. When the suicidal patient is a minor child, the nurse understands that the privilege of confidentiality rests with the:
   a. Minor child
   b. Parents
   c. Nurse
   d. Courts
4. The nurse would institute a no-suicide contract for the patient who:
   a. Is under the influence of drugs
   b. Is socially isolated
   c. Has made previous suicide attempts
   d. Is able to make informed decisions

5. A suicidal patient is prescribed antidepressant therapy. Which of the following medications would the nurse expect to administer to minimize the side effects and improve possible compliance?
   a. Amoxapine (Ascendin)
   b. Imipramine (Tofranil)
   c. Sertraline (Zoloft)
   d. Phenelzine (Nardil)
6. When preparing the suicidal patient for discharge, which of the following statements by the patient would alert the nurse to the possibility of problems after discharge?
   a. "I don't want to burden my family with my problems."
   b. "I've called 2 of my friends who will take turns helping me."
   c. "I'm working on learning how to get along better with others."
   d. "My church has a support group that meets once a week."
7. Which of the following behaviors would be inappropriate for the nurse to implement to reduce the risk for secondary trauma?
   a. Using stress reduction exercises
   b. Internalizing feelings
   c. Maintaining nutrition
   d. Balancing rest and activity
8. When presenting a class about the epidemiology of suicide, the instructor is correct in stating which of the following?
   a. Whites are more likely to complete suicide than nonwhites
   b. Married men and women are more likely to complete suicide
   c. Elderly patients are more likely to be impulsive in their attempts
   d. The risk of suicidal behavior increases with severity of depression

Critical thinking exercises

1. Research the drug, sertraline (Zoloft).
   a. Describe the following:

      Receptor affinity

      Route and dosage

      Half-life (peak effect)

      Adverse reactions

      Contraindications and precautions

   b. Develop a teaching plan for the patient and his family about this drug.

2. Consider this scenario. Caroline is a 19-year-old who visits a busy primary care clinic of a large metropolitan hospital because she has a bad cold and cannot sleep at night. She is triaged to the nurse practitioner who assesses her cold symptoms. Caroline is thin, pale, and tired looking. She is somewhat unkempt, and her hair is pulled back in a pony tail. Her nails and cuticles are chewed, and her leg is in constant motion. Caroline is hostile to the nurse and critical of her every move. When the nurse asks what's bothering her, Caroline yells out, "What's wrong with me? Can't I even get a real doctor? Why do I bother, I'd be better off dead." With that, Caroline breaks down in tears. The nurse sits and waits while Caroline cries. Finally, Caroline begins to talk.

   Caroline tells the nurse that she hasn't been sleeping well for several weeks and her bad cold has made sleep impossible over the last week. All she seems to do is pace in her room at night and wait for morning. Because of lack of sleep, she is very tired and unable to work or go to school. She says that she has no appetite, her stomach stays "tied up in knots," and she has lost several pounds in the last few weeks. She also states that she feels mad all the time and cries easily and often. Lately, all she has been able to do is sit around, but she thinks she may be just worn out from fighting this cold.

The oldest of two children, she lives with her mother and brother. Her father died about a year ago, "took a bottle of sleeping pills." She goes to the local community college and works afternoons as a secretary. She says that she always used to make good grades and has continued to do so until recently. But she has been unable to study well lately, and her grades are falling. When she sits down to study, she finds it impossible to concentrate. She reports that when she has to take a test, her mind goes blank and she cannot remember anything. She says that she has not talked to her teachers, advisor, or mother about her falling grades. She worries that they will be very disappointed in her and that her mother might not give her any more money for school if she finds out.

Caroline tells the nurse that she has always been popular at school with both boys and girls. Her best friend went away to college and she misses her terribly. She says that she had been dating one boy steadily for several years and became pregnant with his child last year. They decided to abort the fetus and since have stopped seeing each other. Caroline says she misses him but has dated other boys since the break up. She comments that she hasn't thought much about the abortion and believes that "having it probably was the right thing to do." She says her social life hasn't been very active lately. When asked what she does when she socializes, Caroline replies, "Same as most kids my age, I guess—hang out and drink."

a. After analyzing this situation, identify possible biopsychosocial etiologies for this patient.

b. Develop a plan of care that addresses this patient's needs.

3. Interview the nurse manager of psychiatric facility to evaluate the methods used to minimize the risk of secondary trauma.

4. As part of a clinical post-conference discussion, your clinical instructor asks you to imagine if a close friend or family member attempted suicide and was successful.

   a. How would you feel?

   b. What strategies would you use to cope with this situation?

35 ▪ *Medical emergencies in psychiatric care*

CHAPTER HIGHLIGHTS

Chapter 35 explores the acute potentially life-threatening medical emergencies that may result from the treatment of psychiatric disorders. It addresses psychopharmacologic agent overdose, neuroleptic malignant syndrome, anticholinergic crisis, serotonin syndrome, and water intoxication. This chapter examines the nurse's role in prevention and early recognition of these conditions and emergency nursing interventions.

Chapter 35 key points include the following:

- Potentially life-threatening medical emergencies may result from or be related to psychiatric treatment.
- The potential for drug overdose and necessity for assessing for toxicity are important for nurses in all settings.
- Identifying the toxic drug is an important part in determining subsequent medical and nursing treatment.
- Supporting the patient's vital functions and assessing vital signs and neurologic status are primary nursing considerations with drug overdose.
- NMS, a potentially life-threatening medical emergency caused by neuroleptic drugs, if left untreated, may be fatal. It is characterized by hyperthermia, muscle rigidity, mental status, and autonomic nervous system changes.
- If NMS is suspected, medications should be withheld and the physician notified immediately.
- Anticholinergic crisis may result from an overdose of muscarinic drugs and also often therapeutic doses of drugs with strong anticholinergic side effects.
- Serotonin syndrome is a toxic effect caused by serotonin reuptake blocking drugs.
- Water intoxication, a severe form of disordered water imbalance in patients with chronic psychiatric disorders, is characterized by abnormally high water intake followed by a rapid drop in serum sodium levels and development of diverse neurologic signs ranging from ataxia to coma.
- Regulating fluid intake and teaching self-monitoring skills are important nursing interventions for patients to control the disorder of water intoxication.

STUDENT ACTIVITIES

Word find

Hidden within the following letter grid are key terms from chapter 35, listed below. The terms may be vertical, horizontal, diagonal, or backward. Circle the words as you find them.

Anticholinergic
Atropine flush
Drug overdose
Diurnal
Hyposthenuria
Lithium
Myoclonus
Myoglobinuria
Polydipsia
Polyuria
Serotonin syndrome
Specific gravity
Toxicity
Tricyclics
Water intoxication

```
T M W H S U L F E N I P O R T A U R I C
R U A S P E C I F I C G R A I M A H V I
I I T E S O D R E V O G U R D Y Y Y I G
C H E B A L T I Y S S R U T H O N P T R
Y T R S E R O T O N I N S Y N D R O M E
A I I U D O U V G I I V S P M G L S Y N
I L A N R U I D E B Y T I C I X O T F I
S D N O T S W A O S A O I O E L C H L L
P Y X L H T I L C Y T A P A R O T E U O
I H I C A R G C I N Z Y N A T B H N I H
D P C O U O X I X D H O P Y H I I U S C
Y T A Y Y B I N O R A T R O P N E R H I
L I L M S E R O T O S C I L C Y C I R T
O O N O I T A C I X O T N I R E T A W N
P S P E C I F I C G R A V I T Y Z I M A
```

Multiple choice

Circle the option that best answers the question.

1. A patient is brought into the emergency room by her husband. The patient is tachycardic with severe hypotension, multifocal premature ventricular contractions, and hyperactive reflexes. The patient has a history of major depressive disorder for which the doctor prescribed a tricyclic antidepressant. The husband says, " I think she took too many pills, that was about 3 hours ago." The nurse would anticipate which of the following?
   a. Hemodialysis
   b. Forced diuresis
   c. Gastric lavage
   d. Intubation
2. A patient's lithium level is 2.7 mEq/L. When assessing this patient, the nurse would expect to find which of the following?
   a. Lethargy
   b. Anorexia
   c. Cogwheel rigidity
   d. Diarrhea
3. A patient who overdosed on benzodiazepines and alcohol is comatose. The nurse anticipates using which agent to reverse the coma?
   a. Flumazenil
   b. Physostigmine
   c. Dantrolene
   d. Bromocriptine
4. The nursing priority for any patient with a suspected drug overdose is:
   a. Patient safety
   b. Patent airway
   c. Neurologic assessment
   d. Cardiac monitoring
5. When teaching a patient about the possibility of NMS, the nurse bases the teaching on the knowledge that this disorder typically occurs with drugs that block which of the following?
   a. Norepinephrine
   b. Serotonin
   c. Histamine
   d. Dopamine

6. When assessing the patient for NMS, the nurse identifies which of the following as the cardinal sign?
   a. Lead pipe rigidity
   b. Hyperthermia
   c. Delirium
   d. Diaphoresis
7. When caring for the patient with NMS, which of the following actions would be inappropriate?
   a. Monitor fluid and hydration status
   b. Protect spastic joints from injury
   c. Withhold neuroleptic agents
   d. Administer anticholinergic agent as ordered
8. A patient is diagnosed with anticholinergic crisis. The physician orders physostigmine 1 mg IV. When administering this drug, the nurse should expect to :
   a. Dilute the drug in 10 cc of normal saline and administer over 10 minutes
   b. Administer by direct injection slowly over 5 minutes
   c. Mix it with 50 cc normal saline and IV piggyback it over 30 minutes
   d. Repeat the dose in 2 hours if no response occurs with the first dose
9. When teaching a patient about serotonin syndrome, the nurse keeps in mind which of the following?
   a. The disorder gradually develops one week after initiating therapy
   b. Hemodialysis is the preferred method of treatment
   c. Extrapyramidal symptoms are common
   d. The disorder generally resolves within 24 hours
10. The nurse observes a patient making frequent trips to the water fountain and carrying a can of soda with him at all times. The nurse suspects water intoxication. Which of the following would help to confirm the nurse's suspicions?
   a. Hyposthenuria
   b. Hypernatremia
   c. Elevated liver enzymes
   d. Diurnal weight loss

Critical thinking exercises

1. Create a decision tree that highlights the emergency nursing care for the patient with a drug overdose. Include appropriate actions for specific types of drug overdoses.

2. Consider this scenario. Gary V., a 52-year-old white man, is a retired computer technician with a long history of chronic paranoid schizophrenia and also a past history of NMS. He lives with his wife who is a teacher. Until recently, Gary attended the day treatment program as the Veteran's Administration Hospital, volunteered at the hospital, bowled weekly, and enjoyed attending hockey games. Gary is compliant with his outpatient medication regimen prescribed, which includes Navane 10 mg, b.i.d., Benadryl 25 mg, b.i.d., and Atenolol 50 mg for hypertension. He is sensitive to trifluoperazine, lithium, fluphenazine, and alprazolam, and NMS developed 2 years ago while he was receiving haloperidol.

   Two weeks ago, Gary became increasingly anxious over a planned airplane trip with his wife to visit his daughter. He began to worry that he might lose control in the airplane and that his symptoms might reappear. Gary's wife brought him to the hospital after Gary reported that the "television was talking to me" and that he heard voices telling him to "kill, kill, kill." Gary was admitted to an inpatient unit for further assessment.

   On admission, Gary is oriented to time, place, and person, and is alert to his surroundings. He is cooperative with the interview process, but pressure of speech is presented. He admits to "hearing voices inside my head telling me to hurt other people" and states that the other patients are "part of the FBI." He denies suicidal thoughts but reports difficulty sleeping for the past two weeks. Temperature is 101, pulse 116, respirations 24/min, and BP 140/90.

   a. Trace the assessment process for this patient to confirm the diagnosis.

   b. Develop a plan of care for this patient that addresses his priority needs.

3. You are assigned to do a class presentation for a group of fellow students about the care of a patient with water intoxication. Develop a lesson plan for the class that integrates the nursing process and biopsychosocial framework.

Suggested readings

Chapter 1

Deutsch, A. 1949. *The mentally ill in America.* New York: Columbia University Press.
This scholarly book describes the care and treatment of the mentally ill from colonial times until the middle of the twentieth century. He traces all the major social issues, the understanding of mental illness, and the treatments that were tried.
Geller, J., & Harris, M. 1994. *Women of the asylum: Voices from behind the walls, 1840–1945.* New York: Anchor Books.
Twenty-six first-person accounts of women who were placed in mental institutions against their will, often by male family members, for holding views or behaving in ways that deviated from the norms of their day are reported. For each era, the accompanying history of both societal and psychiatric standards for women are described.
Hicks, L., Stallmeyer, J., & Coleman, J. 1993. *Role of the nurse in managed care.* Washington, DC: American Nurses Publishing.
This publication gives an introductory overview of managed care, roles for the nurse in managed care, and the future of managed care and nursing. The concept of managed care is defined, historical trends are described, and alternative organizational structures are discussed.
Krauss, J. 1993. *Health care reform: Essential mental health services.* Washington, DC: American Nurses Publishing.
Nursing proposes that mental health reform address the following areas: primary care mental health services, managed care, universal access to a basic mental health benefits package, and structure and financing of the public mental health system for continuous care. Corrective measures are outlined to move the United States a long way toward a comprehensive, coordinated, community-based mental health system that incorporates principles of quality, cost, and managed care.
Pinel, P. 1806. *A treatise on insanity.* New York: Hafner Publishing (reprint translation in 1962).
In this revolutionary book, Philippe Pinel delineates the thoughts that signaled the beginning of the moral treatment era. Through his efforts, the chains were removed from the inmates of the French mental institutions.

Chapter 2

Bachrach, L, Goering, P., & Wasylenki, D., eds. 1994. *Mental health care in Canada.* San Francisco: Jossey-Bass.
This book gives a contemporary view of mental health care in Canada. The Canadian mental health problems and system are compared with the United States system.
Degazon, C. 1994. Ethnic identification, social support and coping strategies among three groups of ethnic African elders. *Journal of Cultural Diversity,* 1(4): 79–85.
This study explored coping strategies as influenced by ethnic and social identity. The results were mixed. In some cases there was a correlation between ethnic identity and coping strategy. Only among Afro-Haitians was coping positively related to social support. (Abstract).
Fabrega, H. 1990. Psychiatric stigma in the classical and medieval period: A review of the literature. *Comprehensive Psychiatry* 31(4): 289–306.

This is a review of material bearing on the question of psychiatric stigma in classical antiquity and the medieval era of Western European societies. The cultural and social factors that contributed to the development of psychiatric stigma are reviewed and analyzed.

Fabrega, H. 1991. Psychiatric stigma in non-Western societies. *Comprehensive Psychiatry* 32(6): 534–51.

Factors bearing on social stigma in persons with psychiatric illnesses are the subject of this review of the literature. The review concentrates on material pertaining to non-Western societies, examining the cultural meanings associated with psychiatric illness. (Abstract).

Hyler, S., Gabbard, G., & Schneider, I. 1989. Homicidal maniacs and narcissistic parasites: Stigmatization of mentally ill persons in the movies. *Hospital and Community Psychiatry* 42(10): 1044–48.

The portrayal of mentally ill persons in movies and television programs has an important and underestimated influence on public perceptions of their condition and care.The authors suggest that mental health professionals can fight this source of stigma by increasing their collaboration with patient advocacy groups, using public information campaigns, and supporting accurate dramatic and documentary depictions of mental illness.

Sharts-Hopko, N. 1996. Health and illness concepts for cultural competence with Japanese clients. *Journal of Cultural Diversity* 3(3): 74–79.

This article discusses health and illness concepts important within the Japanese culture. Self-care and risk behaviors, beliefs and practices related to illness and death, and attitudes toward health professionals are discussed and implications for practice are identified.

Chapter 3

Burdick, M., Stuart, G., & Lewis, L. 1994. Measuring nursing outcomes in a psychiatric setting. *Issues in Mental Health Nursing* 15(2): 137–48.

This article demonstrates the usefulness of the dimensional diagnostic system, NANDA, in identifying specific patient outcomes. Study results indicate that while there were no differences between the two units in the quality of the nursing diagnoses, patient outcomes were addressed more often on the experimental unit.

Lanza, M., Kayne, H., Pattison, I., Hicks, C., & Islam, S. 1994. Predicting violence: Nursing diagnosis versus psychiatric diagnosis. *Nursing Diagnosis* 5(4): 151–57.

This research study demonstrates how a dimensional diagnosis can identify useful clinical data that are not apparent in categorical diagnoses. Two diagnostic assessment systems (Nursing Diagnosis—NANDA and Psychiatric Diagnosis—DSM-III-R) were compared in their ability to predict assaultive behavior.

Mrazek, P., & Haggerty, R., eds. 1994. *Reducing risks for mental disorders: Frontiers for preventive intervention research.* Committee on Prevention of Mental Disorders, Institute of Medicine. Washington, DC: National Academy Press.

A new conceptualization of prevention is the basis of this extensive report by the Committee on Prevention of Mental Disorders whose work was funded by several governmental agencies. In addition to specifying prevention interventions, the report includes a description of five illustrative mental disorders, a discussion of risk and protective factors for the onset of mental disorders, and illustrates preventive intervention research programs. The report also advances a prevention agenda for the next decade.

Malone, J. 1991. The DSM-III-R versus nursing diagnosis: A dilemma in interdisciplinary practice. *Issues in Mental Health Nursing* 12(3): 219–28.

This article discusses the linguistic differences and similarities between the nursing diagnosis classification system and the DSM-III-R psychiatric diagnosis. Dr. Malone emphasizes the importance of using both systems in caring for persons with mental disorders.

Chapter 4

Ganzini, L., Lee, M., Heintz, R., & Bloom, J. 1993. Is the Patient Self-Determination Act appropriate for elderly persons hospitalized for depression. *Journal of Clinical Ethics* 4(1): 46–50, 71–81.

This article is a critique of the Patient Self-Determination Act (PSDA) and its implications for elderly persons who are depressed. The authors argue that the PSDA encourages decisions to be made at a time when these individuals are least capable of autonomous, authentic decision making and most vulnerable to the emotional stresses associated with a discussion.

Gates, M., Schins, I., & Smith, A. 1995. Applying advanced directives regulations in home care agencies. *Home Healthcare Nurse* 14(2): 127–33.

The use of home health care advanced care directives in Michigan were surveyed to determine how the agencies implemented the Self-Determination Act. Of the 108 agencies contacted, 80 completed the survey. The authors identified several areas for improvement.

Milner, S. 1993. An ethical nursing practice model. *Journal of Nursing Administration* 23(3): 22–25.

This article describes a nursing practice model based on five ethical principles that are applied to all aspects of nursing practice. The framework was developed because of the national emphasis on ethical issues and decision making.

Kashka, M., & Keyser, P. 1995. Ethical issues in informed consent and ECT. *Perspectives in Psychiatric Care* 31(2): 15–21.

The ethical concerns of nurses involved with electroconvulsive therapy are explored by using the principles of autonomy and beneficence and analysis of a case study. The authors identify the ethical quandary and provide an update on recommendations for clients giving consent for ECT.

Kinion, E., Jonke, N., & Paradise, N. 1995. Descriptive ethics and neuroleptic dose reduction. *Perspectives in Psychiatric Care* 31(2): 11–14.

This article provides a framework to aid in decision making when psychiatric drugs are decreased in a vulnerable elderly population. A clinical situation is used to illustrate the ethical issues considered in drug reduction.

Parrish, J. 1993. Involuntary use of interventions: Pros and cons. *Innovations and Research in Clinical Services, Community Support, and Rehabilitation* 2(1): 15–22.

This article summarizes some of the principal arguments for and against the use of involuntary interventions disaggregated in terms of the individuals subjected to the interventions, their families, and the mental health system and society at large. It concludes with a recommendation to address the problems cited with the current use of involuntary interventions.

Chapter 5

Abraham, I. L., Fox, J. C., & Cohen, B. T. 1992. Integrating the bio into the biopsychosocial: Understanding and treating biological phenomena in psychiatric-mental health nursing. *Archives of Psychiatric Nursing* 6(5): 296–305.

Theoretically, the discipline of mental health nursing embraces the biopsychosocial sciences, but in actuality there is limited integration of biologic sciences into practice, research, and education. The authors give an overview of how patients were understood from the psychologic and social perspectives, and update the approach by acknowledging the role of neurobiology in understanding the interrelationships between brain, behavior, emotion, and cognition.

Church, O. M. 1991. Parallels and paradoxes: Differentiated nursing practice in psychiatric care. In I. Goertzwen, ed. *Differentiating nursing practice into the twenty-first century.* Selected papers from the 18th Annual Meeting and 1990 Conference of the American Academy of Nursing. Kansas City: American Academy of Nursing.

This article traces psychiatric nursing education from the initiation of training programs in psychiatric hospitals to their acceptance in general nursing programs. The author argues that as psychiatric nursing is integrated into general nursing, the threat of dissolution of the specialty is a constant concern.

Hall, R., & Buckwalter, K. 1990. From ambulance to dedicated unit: Care of institutionalized elderly with behavioral problems. *Archives of Psychiatric Nursing* 4(1): 3–11.

This article provides an historical overview of the care of older persons with behavioral problems, from the almshouses of the early twentieth century to the dedicated care units of today. The role of the psychiatric nurse in relation to the need for more mental health programming and changes in reimbursement mechanisms for the institutionalized elderly is examined. (Abstract).

Harper, M., & Grau, L. 1994. State of the art in geropsychiatric nursing. *Journal of Psychosocial Nursing* 32(4): 7–12.

This article summarizes the prevalence of mental disorders among the elderly, emphasizes viewing the family as a patient, and discusses the underdiagnosis and underuse of mental health services.

Kerr, J., & MacPhail, J. 1991. *Canadian nursing: Issues and perspectives.* St. Louis: Mosby-Year Book.

This book presents an overview of Canadian nursing, including the development of the profession of nursing, generation of nursing knowledge, issues related to delivery of care, and an overview of nursing education.

Richards, B. 1994. Geropsychiatric nursing: Present issues and future challenges. *Nursing Clinics of North America* 29(1): 49–56.

The article examines the history and development of geropsychiatric nursing. The nature and scope of practice is characterized as collaborative and interdisciplinary because of the complexity, diversity, and dissimilarity of elderly persons.

Scahill, L. 1991. Nursing diagnosis vs. goal-oriented treatment planning in inpatient child psychiatry. *Image: Journal of Nursing Scholarship* 23(2): 95–98.

In an inpatient unit, timely evaluation, stabilization, and discharge of children requires multidisciplinary teamwork. This article considers the merit of nursing diagnosis in child inpatient psychiatry, which carries some risk of creating parallel systems of care and isolating nurses from the treatment team.

Chapter 6

Jewell, J., & Sullivan, E. 1996. Application of nursing theories in health education. *Journal of the American Psychiatric Nurses Association* 2(3): 79–85.

This article demonstrates how the theories of Hildegarde Peplau and Dorothea Orem can be applied to two different health education groups. The utility of these two theories to guide nursing practice is supported.

Hopton, J. 1996. Reconceptualizing the theory-practice gap in mental health nursing. *Nurse Education Today* 16(3): 227–32.

This paper identifies the key problems in bridging the gap between theory and practice in the education of mental health nurses and proposes a strategy for overcoming these problems, proposing a unified model of clinical nursing practice, nurse education, and user involvement, which would place nurse educators at the forefront of the reform of mental health services.

Keddy, B. 1996. A feminist critique of psychiatric nursing discourse. *Issues in Mental Health Nursing* 17(4): 381–91.

This theoretical research explores the discourse, language, texts, and practices that are part of the world of psychiatric nursing. The author argues that psychiatric nursing "science" has developed from the work of nursing theorists and researchers in an attempt to raise the status of nursing. The results have been that this knowledge wields power.

Ziegler, S., ed. 1993. *Theory-directed nursing practice.* New York: Springer.

This book is an excellent supplement to the theory discussions in this chapter. Nine theoretical models are explained and applied to patient situations.

Chapter 7

Andreasen, N. C. 1984. *The broken brain: The biological revolution in psychiatry.* New York: Harper & Row.

Although somewhat older, this readable work of nonfiction provides an introduction to the basics of biologic psychiatry, including the history of its development. The historical content also provides ample evidence that though the "biologic revolution" is often considered to be recent, it actually is quite old.

Andreasen, N. C., & Black, D. W. 1995. *Introductory textbook of psychiatry,* 2nd ed. Washington, DC: American Psychiatric Press.

Chapter 4 of this textbook provides more description and application of laboratory tests, including neuroimaging techniques, for readers interested in these areas. In addition, chapter 5 examines the neurobiology of mental illness with another review of the structure and function of the brain as it applies to psychiatry. Other chapters in this textbook include biologic hypotheses of each major psychiatric disorder.

Betrus, P. A., & Elmore, S. K. 1991. Seasonal affective disorder, part I: A review of the neural mechanisms for psychosocial nurses. *Archives of Psychiatric Nursing* (5): 357–64.
While reviewing the pathways of the suprachiasmatic nucleus as related to the pineal body and secretion of melatonin, this article applies basic knowledge in neuroscience to understanding current hypotheses of seasonal affective disorder.
DeArmond, S. J., Fusco, M. M., & Dewey, M. M. 1995. *Structure of the human brain: A photographic atlas,* 4th ed. New York: Oxford.
On facing pages, this atlas presents schematic drawings with descriptive identifications directly opposite pictures of actual brain tissue. Initially covering gross brain anatomy, the presentations incorporate computer-assisted brain imaging techniques of a variety of cross-sections throughout the spinal cord, brain stem, cerebrum, and cerebellum, allowing the reader to visualize all of the subcortical structures and nuclei.
Elmore, S. K. 1991. Seasonal affective disorder, part II: Phototherapy, an expanded role of the psychosocial nurse. *Archives of Psychiatric Nursing* (5): 365–72.
Within the context of seasonal affective disorder, this article reviews circadian rhythm and REM sleep changes in affective disorders. Readers are provided with an example of how biologic knowledge may be applied to the development of a treatment such as phototherapy.
Hyman, S. E., & Nestler, E. J. 1993. *The molecular foundations of psychiatry.* Washington, DC: American Psychiatric Press.
This book is an excellent resource for more indepth information concerning synaptic transmission, neurotransmitters, neuromodulators, and psychiatric genetics. Complete with diagrams, tables summarizing complex information, and sections marked for the advanced reader, even the novice can use this text to easily find, acquire, and integrate current research and hypotheses into an understanding of the basis of biologic psychiatry.
Laraia, M. 1995. *Biology, brain and behavior: A psychiatric nursing perspective.* American Psychiatric Nurses Association Slide Kit. Belle Mead, NJ: Excerpta Medica.
This kit of 45 slides and related text begins with an excellent review of neuroanatomy and basic neurophysiology.
Nihart, M. A. 1993. The development of neurotransmitter systems. *Journal of Child and Adolescent Psychiatric and Mental Health Nursing* 6(3): 23–24.
Not all neurotransmitter systems and pathways develop at the same rate. This article reviews the neuronal growth and development of some of the major neurotransmitter systems, including dopamine, serotonin, norepinephrine, and acetylcholine.
Society for Neuroscience. 1990. *Brain facts: A primer on the brain and nervous system.* Washington, DC: Author.
This 31-page booklet provides an illustrated review of the structure and function of the brain, including the neuron, neurotransmitters, and neural development. Also covered are the integral workings of the human responses of sensation and perception, learning and memory, and movement.
Schindler, L. W. 1990. *Understanding the immune system* NIH Publication No. 90-529. Rockville, MD: U.S. Department of Health and Human Services.
This government publication contains an overview of the anatomy, cells, secretions, and response of the immune system.Numerous pictures and schematics illustrate the complex nature of immune function.

Chapter 8

Bezchlibnyk-Butler, K. Z., & Jeffries, J. J. 1995. *Clinical handbook of psychotropic drugs,* 5th ed. Seattle: Hogrefe & Huber.
This spiral-bound reference provides quick access to information regarding all medications used in psychiatry as well as psychoactive substances of abuse.
Harris, J. E. 1992. Psychopharmacology. In J. A. Malone, ed. *Schizophrenia: Handbook for Clinical Care,* pp. 39–68. Thorofare, NJ: Slack.
From indications to side-effect management, this book chapter provides a comprehensive review of medications used in the treatment of schizophrenia. Both standard neuroleptic treatment and atypical antipsychotics are covered.

Najarian, S. P. 1995. Family experience with positive client response to clozapine. *Archives of Psychiatric Nursing* (9): 11–21.

The paper illustrates the effects that improvement of symptoms can have on those who are close to the individual receiving the medication.

Schatzberg, A. F., & Nemeroff, M. D. 1995. *Textbook of psychopharmacology.* Washington, DC: American Psychiatric Press.

For more advanced information or as a reference, this work provides the most comprehensive application of current knowledge, theory, and research in psychopharmacology that is currently available in a textbook for the treatment of psychiatric disorders.

Valente, S. M. 1991. Electroconvulsive therapy. *Archives of Psychiatric Nursing,* 5: 223–28.

This article reviews current research and procedural information regarding electroconvulsive therapy. It includes case examples and illustrates nursing's critical involvement in patient education, advocacy, and monitoring.

Wolfe, B. E. 1995. Dimensions of response to antidepressant agents in bulimia nervosa: A review. *Archives of Psychiatric Nursing* (9): 111–21.

Examining sixteen placebo-controlled treatments, this review provides a strong example of the need for alternative measures for treatment outcomes related to psychotropic medication. Rating scales and other measures typically used are addressed, but this author illustrates that other areas of impact by medications on an individual's life are rarely assessed.

Chapter 9

Fowler, J. 1994. A welcome focus on a key relationship: Using Peplau's model in palliative care. *Professional Nurse* 10(3): 194–97.

Peplau's model of the key stages that mark that the nurse-patient relationship may be used in palliative care. This model can be used for models of grief, such as Murray Parkes and Kübler-Ross. Both grief theories are based on the belief that the nurse-patient relationship determines whether or not the patient's experience of illness is a positive one.

Fosbinder, D. 1994. Patient perceptions of nursing care: An emerging theory of interpersonal competence. *Journal of Advanced Nursing* 20(6): 1085–93.

This article reports results from a qualitative research project that identified elements of interpersonal competence among nurses from their respective patients. Four major processes emerged from the data to provide the framework for the themes: translating, getting to know you, establishing trust, and going the extra mile.

Rogers, S. 1996. Facilitative affiliation: Nurse-client interactions that enhance healing. *Issues in Mental Health Nursing* 17(3): 171–84.

This article supports the effectiveness of the therapeutic relationship in facilitating the following patient outcomes: achievement of client goals, satisfaction with nursing care, comfort, growth, and enhanced healing. The author combines the concepts of facilitation and affiliation to describe the essence of the nurse-patient interaction.

Scott, A., & Dumas, R. 1995. Personal space boundaries: Clinical applications in psychiatric mental health nursing. *Perspectives in Psychiatric Care* 31(3): 14–19.

These authors present another way of looking at boundaries. They define personal space boundaries, arguing that these concepts can be applied in the clinical setting to heighten the nurse's boundary awareness and provide a perspective of intervention that incorporates the interactive effects of cognition, affect, behavior, and spirituality on human experience and behavior.

Sines, D. 1994. The arrogance of power: A reflection on contemporary mental health nursing practice. *Journal of Advanced Nursing* 20(5): 894–903.

This article explores the role of contemporary mental health nursing and challenges practitioners to acknowledge the influence that power relationships have on therapeutic practice and client outcomes.

Chapter 10

Mezey, M., Mitty, E., & Ramsey, G. 1997. Assessment of decision-making capacity: Nursing's role. *Journal of Gerontological Nursing* 23 (3): 28–35, 50–56.

This article provides another perspective in using mental status assessment. The authors argue that the mental status assessment test cannot be the sole criterion for determining decision-making ability.
Eppard, J., & Anderson, J. 1995. Emergency psychiatric assessment: The nurse, psychiatrist, and counselor roles during the process. *Journal of Psychosocial Nursing and Mental Health Services.* 22(10): 17–23, 42–44.
The authors describe the roles of psychiatric nurses, psychiatrists, and counselors, exploring the differences in their perceptions of teamwork, responsibility, role expectation, and in connecting with clients.
Cardell, R., Horton-Deutsch, S. 1994. A model for assessment of inpatient suicide potential. *Archive of Psychiatric Nursing* 8(6): 366–72.
Psychiatric inpatient suicides have unique characteristics compared with suicides that occur on an outpatient basis. The authors argue that a number of factors play a role in determining whether patients will kill themselves in the hospital.

Chapter 11

Merwin, E., & Mauch, A. 1995. Psychiatric nursing outcome research. The state of the *science. Archives in Psychiatric Nursing* 9(6): 311–31.
The authors review the nursing literature from 1989 to 1994 and report on the state of outcome research in psychiatric nursing. They discuss strategies for increasing the quantity and quality of psychiatric nursing outcome research.
Sainfort, F., Becker, M., & Diamond, R. 1996. Judgments of quality of life of individuals with severe mental disorders: Patient self report versus provider perspectives. *American Journal of Psychiatry* 153(4): 497–502.
This study is an example of interdisciplinary collaboration of nurses with other disciplines. The authors concluded that mental health services should address a wide range of needs reflecting different aspects of quality of life perceived important by different patients.
Idvall, E., Rooke, L., & Hamrin, E. 1997. Quality indicators in clinical nursing: A review of the literature. *Journal of Advanced Nursing* 25(1): 6–17.
The article is a report on a literature review of clinical indicators used in nursing. This review revealed that there is an uncertainty regarding the use of terms such as indicators, standard, norm, criteria, and aspects of care.

Chapter 12

Bowles, K., & Naylor, M. 1996. Nursing intervention classification systems. *Image: Journal of Nursing Scholarship* 28(4): 302–8.
This article analyzes the features, development, and research of the Omaha system, the Iowa nursing intervention classification, and the home health care classification and provides a critical review of the unique components of each.
McCloskey, J., & Bulechek, G. 1996. *Nursing interventions classification NIC.* St. Louis: Mosby.
This book contains a validated and coded taxonomic structure in which all 433 interventions are located according to their relationships with similar interventions. The interventions have also been linked to nursing diagnoses according to the North American Nursing Diagnosis Association NANDA.

Chapter 13

American Association for Partial Hospitalization. 1994. *Overview of the partial hospitalization industry.* Alexandria, VA: AAPH Publications.
This publication contains tables and analyses of partial hospitalization programs. It compares programs by lengths of stay, population served, and the full range of program organization, management, and financial variables. It also presents trends by comparing data gathered in 1992 and 1994.
Evashwick, C., & Weiss, L. 1987. *Managing the continuum of care.* Rockville, MD: Aspen.

This book examines the issues and problems administrators and clinicians face in creating a comprehensive, integrated continuum of care. It presents concepts and general lessons of operating a continuum of care.

Flynn, A. M., & Kilgallen, M. E. 1993. Case management: A multidisciplinary approach to the evaluation of cost and quality standards. *Journal of Nursing Care Quality* 8(1): 58–66.

This article describes a multidisciplinary case management model that addresses cost and quality by unifying resources and expert clinical knowledge through a unit care map. The care map defines the role and responsibilities of the clinician and the patient for more efficient use of therapeutic time.

Joint Commission on the Accreditation of Healthcare Organizations. 1994. *Accreditation manual for mental health, chemical dependency, and mental retardation/ developmental disabilities services.* Oakbrook Terrace, IL: Author.

This manual is used as a tool for behavioral health care providers seeking accreditation. The JCAHO manual defines the function of the continuum of care. Additionally, JCAHO sets standards based on outcomes for various components of the continuum of care.

Lehman, A. F., Scott, J. E., Dixon, L. B., & Thompson, J. W. 1995. Schizophrenia: Treatment outcomes research. *Schizophrenia Bulletin* 21(4).

The schizophrenia PORT study examines outcomes of treatments for schizophrenia and seeks to lay out an agenda for available research knowledge to be transferred into practices and for future research into outcomes.

Chapter 14

The Expert Consensus Guidelines Series: Treatment of schizophrenia. *Journal of Clinical Psychiatry,* Supplement 12B, 57, 1996.

This supplement provides an excellent overview of current thinking on the treatment of schizophrenia. It includes guides for patients and families as well as treatment issues and drug doses and side effects.

Budd, R., Hughes, C., & Smith, J. 1996. Health beliefs and compliance with antipsychotic medication. *British Journal of Clinical Psychiatry* 3(5): 393–97.

This research article uses the Health Belief Model to explain compliance with antipsychotic medication. The use of one of the nursing models provides an opportunity to see how it translates in other fields.

Chouvardas, J. 1996. The symbolic and the literal in schizophrenic language. *Perspectives in Psychiatric Care* 32(2): 20–22.

This short article looks at how schizophrenics use metaphors, poetry, and symbols in their language. It provides possibilities for nurses to think about to enhance their therapeutic effectiveness with these patients.

Chapter 15

Blise, M. 1995. Everything I learned, I learned from patients: Radical positive reframing. *Journal of Psychosocial Nursing and Mental Health Services* 33(12): 18–25, 40–41.

Reframing allows a situation to be viewed in a different way. Reframing can assist the patient to develop less threatening explanations for paranoid delusion. This article shows how patients can be taught to present their delusions as their feelings, not as actual events.

Duff, A. 1996. Case study of a female client on a regional secure unit. *Journal of Advanced Nursing* 23(4): 771–75.

This article reports on a single case study of a 32-year-old female inpatient with a psychiatric disorder. It is useful for planning care to decrease maladaptive behaviors and symptoms and for increasing positive behaviors.

Keltner, J. 1995. Psychopharmacology update. Risperidone: The search for a better antipsychotic. *Perspectives in Psychiatric Care* 31(1): 30–33.

In the regular column, Psychopharmacology Update, an overview of the new atypical antipsychotic, risperidone, is given. Action, effectiveness, dosage, and side effects are discussed.

O'Connell, K. 1995. Schizoaffective disorder: A case study. *Journal of Psychosocial Nursing and Mental Health Services* 33(10): 35–40, 42–43.

In a case study of an elderly patient, the author provides and reviews diagnosis and treatment of schizoaffective disorder. She argues that the elderly client presents special challenges and recommends case management as important.

Wright, J., Burgess, A., Bugress, A., et al. 1995. Investigating stalking crimes. *Journal of Psychosocial Nursing and Mental Health Services* 33(9): 38–43.

This article identifies three types of stalkers as the nondomestic stalker who may know the target through social contact or from a random meeting in a public place, the domestic stalker who may be known to the target and had a close personal relationship with the target, and the erotomania stalker whose target is typically a public figure. Stalking is conceptualized on a continuum from nondelusional to delusional behavior. (Abstract modified).

Chapter 16

Irvin, S. M. 1997. Treatment of depression with outpatient electroconvulsive therapy. *AORN Journal* 65(3): 573–78, 581–82.

This article explains the use of ECT in the treatment of depression. Successful performance of outpatient ECT requires collaboration by skilled perioperative nurses, psychiatrists, anesthesia care providers, affected individuals, and family members.

Heifner, C. 1997. The male experience of depression. *Perspectives in psychiatric care* 33(2): 10–18.

The article reports on a qualitative study of men's experience of depression. Beliefs about being male are challenged by the illness and challenge the process of treatment and recovery.

Pollack, L. E. 1996. Inpatients with bipolar disorder: Their quest to understand. *Journal of Psychosocial Nursing* 34(6): 19–24.

The article explores the quest to understand how to live with the recurrent major mental illness of bipolar disorder. Individual and group work with this population needs to include discussion of how to obtain self-management information when out of the hospital, potential barriers that may be encountered in the pursuit of such information, and adaptive and maladaptive responses to barriers.

Flenniken, M. C. 1997. Psychotropic prescriptive patterns among nurse practitioners in nonpsychiatric settings. *Journal of the American Academy of Nurse Practitioner* 9(3): 117–21.

This study explores mental health care treatment among primary care nurse practitioners. The need for continuing education in psychopharmacology among primary care nurse practitioners is highlighted.

Grant. S. M., Hardin, S. B., Pesut, D. J., & Hardin, T. 1997. Psychological evaluations, referrals, and follow up of adolescents after their exposure to Hurricane Hugo. *Journal of Child and Adolescent Psychiatric Nursing* 10(1): 7–16.

This study describes the psychological evaluations, referrals, and follow-up assessments made by nurse practitioners and a nurse psychotherapist of adolescents in two South Carolina high schools who experienced Hurricane Hugo. The authors propose a model suggesting that adolescent appraisal of stress and crisis is a critical issue to consider when intervening with adolescents who are exposed to major stressors.

Warren, B. J. 1997. Depression, stressful life events, social support, and self esteem in middle class African American women. *Archives of Psychiatric Nursing* 11(3): 107–17.

This article describes an exploratory study that examined relationships between depression, stressful life events, social support, and self-esteem in middle class African-American women, aged 20 to 35 years. Results showed a positive relationship between depression and stressful life events and a negative relationship between and social support.

Chapter 17

Burgess, A., Hartman, C., & Clements, P. 1995. Biology of memory and childhood trauma. *Journal of Psychosocial Nursing and Mental Health Services* 33(3): 16–26.

The authors review the effects of trauma on the limbic system and the resulting neurohormonal changes. The concept of trauma learning is presented, followed by case studies dramatizing the didactic information.

Cooper, C. 1995. Psychiatric stress debriefing. *Journal of Psychosocial Nursing and Mental Health Services* 33(5): 21–25.

The author presents a strategy for psychiatric staffs to use in processing patient assaults and suicides. This technique, called critical incident stress debriefing, is compared with the psychological autopsy.
Glod, C., & McEnany, G. 1995. The neurobiology of posttraumatic stress disorder. *Journal of the American Psychiatric Nurses Association* 1(6): 196–99.
The authors present an excellent review of studies related to brain abnormalities among patients who have PTSD. The article concludes with a discussion of implications for nursing practice.
Godbey, K., & Courage, M. 1994. Stress-management program: Intervention in nursing student performance anxiety. *Archives of Psychiatric Nursing* VIII(3): 190–99.
The authors studied a six-week stress management program among student nurses whose anxiety affected academic performance. Results indicated that the program was helpful in increasing self-esteem, decreasing anxiety, and improving grades.
Laraia, M. 1991. Biological correlates of panic disorder with agoraphobia: Practice perspectives for nurses. *Archives of Psychiatric Nursing* V(6): 373–81.
The author reviews the literature about panic disorder, including biologic theories based on laboratory tests and positron emission tomography studies. A review of applicable psychopharmacology is included. Implications for nursing practice are suggested.

Chapter 18

Linehan, M. 1993. *Cognitive-behavioral treatment of borderline personality disorder.* New York: Guilford Press.
This book is highly recommended for anyone who cares for someone with a BPD. Dr. Linehan conceptualizes BPD within a biosocial framework that focuses on emotional dysregulation.
Selzer, J. 1992. Borderline omnipotence in pathological gambling. *Archives of Psychiatric Nursing* 6(4): 215–18.
Borderline omnipotence in pathologic gambling is examined, including psychodynamics of omnipotence, a theory of the patient's use of omnipotence in pathologic gambling, and the effects of the omnipotence on the treatment and recovery of the pathologic gambler. Assessment, staff education, and the need for individualized treatment for the pathologic gambler are discussed.
Stein, K. 1996. Affect instability in adults with a borderline personality disorder. *Archives of Psychiatric Nursing* 10(1): 32–40.
This article describes a study of the pattern of mood instability in adults with BPD. Twenty-eight individuals were studied for mood fluctuations.The findings showed that BPD subjects experienced higher levels of unpleasant moods and greater short-term fluctuations in unpleasant moods than the asymptomatic subjects. Even though the sample was small, the findings support the association of mood instability with BPD.
Warmbrodt, L., Hardy, R., & Chrisman, S. 1996. Understanding trichotillomania. *Journal of Psychosocial Nursing* 34(12): 11–15.
This article explains trichotillomania, including the description, prevalence, etiologic issues, and its relationship to other disorders. The authors explain the nursing management of these patients and describe approaches to care. Client education and self-monitoring are emphasized.

Chapter 19

Tabora, B., & Flaskerud, J. 1994. Depression among Chinese Americans: A review of the literature. *Issues in Mental Health Nursing* 15(6): 569–84.
This article gives a general review of the literature on depression among Chinese Americans to clarify misconceptions, to increase knowledge of research on depression that has been done on one specific Asian-American group, and to set a direction for future nursing research and intervention. (Abstract).
Feldman, M., & Eisendrath, S. 1996. *The spectrum of factitious disorders.* Washington, DC: American Psychiatric Press.

This book presents a useful discussion of factitious disorders providing an overview of the disorders from a historical and contemporary perspective. Psychological and physical factitious disorders are distinguished from each other.

Hulme, P. 1996. Somatization in Hispanics. *Journal of Psychosocial Nursing and Mental Health Services* 34(3): 33–37.

Major psychological disorders are found universally, but their form and content are modified by culture. The expression of psychosocial distress is largely shaped by cultural values and beliefs. Preliminary research indicates Hispanics are more likely to somatize than Anglos when experiencing psychosocial disorders of psychosocial distress. This article supports the need for an assessment for specific somatic problems for Hispanic women. Somatic symptoms such as headache, backache, and gastrointestinal discomfort may signify an underlying depression that is being expressed through physical sensations.

Chapter 20

Corcoran, M., & Gitlin, L. N. 1991. Environmental influences on behavior of the elderly with delirium: Principles for intervention in the home. *Physical and Occupational Therapy in Geriatrics* 9 (3/4): 5–22.

This article uses the environmental model developed by Barris and colleagues in developing twelve intervention principles for altering the home environment of elderly patients with delirium to reduce their oversensitivity to stimuli and establish a safe environment. Intervention techniques are illustrated by case examples.

Foreman, M. 1986. Reliability and validity of mental status questionnaires in elderly hospitalized patients. *Nursing Research* 3(6): 216–20.

This article reports on a study of the comparative reliability and validity of the Short Portable Mental Status Questionnaire, the Mini-Mental State Examination, and the Cognitive Capacity Screening Examination using a study sample of 66 elderly patients on general medical-surgical units. Content validity, criterion validity, instrument sensitivity, and internal consistency reliability were examined for the three instruments.

Liptzin, B., & Levkoff, S. E. 1992. An empirical study of delirium subtypes. *British Journal of Psychiatry* 16(1): 843–45.

This study assessed the behaviors indicative of delirium in 325 older patients who were admitted to the hospital for acute medical problems. Four subtypes were identified: hyperactive, hypoactive, mixed, and neither. The authors suggest the hyperactive group may be more likely to receive medical and nursing attention, thereby shortening length of stay and improving chances of survival.

Sorbi, S. 1993. Molecular genetics of Alzheimer's disease. *Aging Clinical and Experimental Research* 5: 417–25.

This study presented new approaches and results in molecular biology that have provided new insights into possible etiologic mechanisms of familial Alzheimer's disease.

Zarit, S. H., & Whitlatch, C. J. 1992. Institutional placement: Phases of the transition. *The Gerontologist* 32(5): 665–72.

The study reviewed the effects of placing delirium patients in institutionalized care on a sample of caregivers. Consistent with the stress process model, institutional placement relieved relatives of the primary stressors of caregiving (e.g., feelings of overload, tension, and tiredness), whereas other indicators of stress remained unchanged.

Chapter 21

Halmi, K. A., ed. 1992. *Psychobiology and treatment of anorexia nervosa and bulimia nervosa.* Washington, DC: American Psychiatric Press.

In-depth and applicable knowledge related to diagnosis, genetics, outcome studies, neurobiology, and other treatments for eating disorders are provided in an easily readable and understandable manner.

Chapter 22

Alcoholics Anonymous World Services, Inc. 1976. *Alcoholics Anonymous.* New York: Author.

Since 1939, this book has been the blueprint of a recovery program suggested by Alcoholics Anonymous. It describes the program and how it works, and has first-person accounts of individual recovery from alcoholism.

Beck, A. Wright, F. D., Newman, C. F., & Liese, B. S. 1993. *Cognitive therapy of substance abuse.* New York: Guilford Press.

This book describes a methodology of addressing substance abuse disorders through use of cognitive therapy techniques. It is practical and has helpful dialogues of therapist-patient interactions.

Finke, L., Williams J., & Stanley, R. 1996. Nurses referred to a peer assistance program for alcohol and drug problems. *Archives of Psychiatric Nursing* X(5): 319–24.

Interesting study results regarding 221 nurses referred to a state nursing organization peer assistance program describing nurse characteristics, chemical substance use, and program participation of these registered nurses who engaged in peer treatment program for substance abuse. Emphasizes the role of nursing education in overall prevention of alcohol and drug problems.

Kitchens, J. A. 1991. *Understanding and treating codependence.* Englewood Cliffs, NJ: Prentice Hall.

This book reviews several models of codependence and presents clear interventions in the context of group treatment for this problem, with pertinent clinical examples to illustrate issues.

Lowinson, J. H., Ruiz, P., Millman, R. R., & Langrod, J. G., eds. 1992. *Substance abuse: A comprehensive textbook.* Baltimore: Williams & Wilkins.

A comprehensive medical textbook written by leaders in treatment of substance abuse disorders covering historical and legal perspectives, etiology of substance abuse, abusable substances, and assessment and treatment approaches. Particular emphasis is placed on special populations and policy issues.

Marlatt, G. A., & Gordon, 1985. *Relapse prevention.* New York: Guilford Press.

This textbook describes a model of addiction and of relapse prevention. It outlines a program of relapse prevention groups based on cognitive and skill-training intervention.

Miller, W. R., & Rollnick, S. 1991. *Motivational interviewing: Preparing people to change addictive behavior.* New York: Guilford Press.

This book outlines a process for increasing motivation for changing addictive behavior, discussing the stages that patients go through in making changes together with appropriate interventions for each stage. Most importantly, it discusses ways of enhancing commitment to recovery without getting into traditional power struggles and nontherapeutic interventions with those who are resistant to change.

Monti, P. M., Abrams, D. B., & Cooney, N. L. 1989. *Treating alcohol dependence.* New York: Guilford Press.

This book outlines a comprehensive treatment program based on a cognitive-social learning theory approach to substance abuse. It teaches skills that enhance ways to stop use and provides outlines for teaching such interpersonal skills as drink refusal, giving and getting criticism, enhancing social support networks, and improving intrapersonal skills, such as managing thoughts about alcohol, problem-solving, relaxation training, and anger management.

Vanicelli, M. 1989. *Removing the roadblocks: Group psychotherapy with substance abusers and family members.* New York: Guilford Press.

This book discusses basic group therapy techniques and outlines their specific use with substance abusers and with family members. It is readable and provides an excellent background in leading early recovery, abstinence-focused groups.

Wallace, J. 1989. *Writing: The alcoholism papers.* Newport, RI: Edgehill Publications.

This is a collection of the writing of a well-respected therapist in the field of alcoholism treatment. This is an excellent background reader for substance abuse treatment issues.

Chapter 23

Anch, A. M., Browman, C. P., Mitler, M. M., & Walsh, J. K. 1988. *Sleep: A scientific perspective.* Englewood Cliffs, NJ: Prentice Hall.

This text is intended for students as well as allied health professionals. This is an excellent starting point for the beginning inquiries into the basic science of sleep. Landmark research is well synthesized.

Carskadon, M. A., ed. 1993. *Encyclopedia of sleep and dreaming.* New York: Macmillan.

The encyclopedia is organized alphabetically with topics ranging from hard science to whimsical anecdotes. Everything from arousal mechanisms to pajamas are covered.

Ferber, R. F. 1985. *Solve your child's sleep problems.* New York: Simon & Schuster.

This is an excellent reference for parents and health care workers who are confounded by children's sleep problems. There are detailed steps for parents when children have difficulty falling asleep on their own, not staying in bed, and enuresis.

Kryger, M. H., Roth, T., & Dement, W. C., eds. 1994. *Principles and practice of sleep medicine,* 2nd ed. Philadelphia: Saunders.

This is the most comprehensive reference in the field of sleep medicine. Themes are drawn from a variety of disciplines. The book is divided into two parts. The first part focuses on the basic science of sleep. The second section focuses on clinical considerations: abnormal sleep, disorders of chronobiology, insomnia, primary disorders of daytime somnolence, parasomnias, sleep breathing disorders, medical disorders, psychiatric disorders, and methodology.

Monk, T. H., & Folkard, S. 1992. *Making shiftwork tolerable.* Bristol, PA: Taylor & Francis.

This is an easy-to-read compilation of research on shiftwork. The intended audience is the shift worker. Discussions include topics from the field of chronobiology, the latest theories about the effects of shift work, and research on coping strategies.

Chapter 24

Beck, J. 1995. Hypoactive sexual desire disorder: An overview. *Journal of Consulting and Clinical Psychology* 63(6): 919–27.

This article reviews the current state of knowledge about hypoactive sexual desire disorder. It reviews diagnostic issues, including prevalence estimates. Throughout, areas where additional work is needed are highlighted.

Frable, D. 1997. Gender, racial, ethnic, sexual, and class identities. *Annual Review of Psychology* 4(8): 139–62.

This chapter summarizes how people create and negotiate their gender, racial, ethnic, sexual, and class identities. Research suggests that these are fluid, multidimensional, personalized social construction that reflect the individual's current context and sociohistorical cohort.

Gitlin, M. 1994. Psychotropic medications and their effects on sexual function: Diagnosis, biology, and treatment approaches. *Journal of Clinical Psychiatry* 55(9): 406–13.

The author reviews case reports, case series, and animal studies on the topics of the effect of psychiatric disorders on sexual functioning, the biology of sex, rates of sexual dysfunction associated with each medication class, and treatment approaches when these side effects occur.

Hyde, J. & Kavoussi, R. 1996. *Understanding human sexuality.* New York: McGraw-Hill Book Company.

This undergraduate textbook can support knowledge in human sexuality.

Ogden, J. & Ward, E. 1995. Help-seeking behavior in sufferers of vaginismus. *Sexual and Marital Therapy* 10(1): 23–30.

The authors examined help-seeking behaviors among 89 vaginismic females and explores their general experiences of professional intervention. Results showed that there is a widespread dissatisfaction with professional interventions for this problem.

O'Farrell, T., Choquette, K., Cutter, H., & Birchler, G. 1997. Sexual satisfaction and dysfunction in marriages of male alcoholics: Comparison with nonalcoholic maritally conflicted and nonconflicted couples. *Journal of Studies of Alcohol* 58(1): 91–99.

This study examined the contribution of alcoholism and marital conflict to male alcoholics' sexual problems. This study implicates marital conflict and alcoholism are major contributing factors to the rates of impotence.

Chapter 25

Canino, I. A., & Spurlock, J. S. 1994. *Culturally diverse children and adolescents: Assessment, diagnosis and treatment planning.* New York: Guilford.

Rather than breaking chapters down by ethnic groups, this volume provides an integrative approach to culturally sensitive assessment and treatment of children and adolescents, primarily on African-American, Latino, Asian-American, and American-Indian children. The strength of the book is its detailed approach to history-taking and diagnosis, including a chapter on DSM IV and the unique aspects of applying this diagnostic system to minority youth.

Coleman, M., & Ganong, L. H. 1988. *Bibliotherapy with stepchildren.* Springfield, IL: Charles C. Thomas.

This comprehensive guide to 265 books is designed to address concerns of children in stepfamilies. In an exhaustive review, the authors identify the focus of each book (i.e., stepmother, stepfather, stepsiblings) and evaluate each one for quality and themes addressed. The book is designed for professionals, educators, and parents.

Combrinck-Graham, L., ed. 1989. *Children in family contexts: Perspectives on treatment.* New York: Guilford.

This edited volume covers the gamut of common stressors of childhood and adolescence and includes in-depth chapters on adoption, chronic illness, remarriage, parental alcoholism, family violence, poverty, immigration, out-of-home placement, and the threat of nuclear war.

Dunn, J., & Plomin, R. 1990. *Separate lives: Why siblings are so different.* New York: Basic Books.

This book is written by two of the leading researchers who are exploring the relative contributions of genetics versus the environment in child development. The book examines the question of why siblings who share roughly 50 percent of the same genes sometimes develop so differently. The impacts of genes, parental behavior, peers, sibling relationships, and chance events are examined.

Forman, S. G. 1993. *Coping skills interventions for children and adolescents.* San Francisco: Jossey-Bass.

This handy volume outlines a variety of interventions for increasing coping skills in children and adolescents, including relaxation techniques, social skills training, problem solving, assertiveness, decreasing irrational beliefs, success-oriented thinking, and behavioral self-control.

Gibbs, J. T., & Huang, L. N., eds. 1989. *Children of color: Psychological interventions with minority youth.* San Francisco: Jossey-Bass.

This book addresses the special needs of minority children and adolescents with psychological and behavioral problems, emphasizing the impact of poverty, discrimination, and immigration on the development of minority youth.

Rolf, J., Masten, A. S., Cicchetti, D., et al., eds. 1990. *Risk and protective factors in the development of psychopathology.* Cambridge: Cambridge University Press.

This scientific volume provides an extensive review of research on risk and protective factors for psychiatric disorders. Although it covers a wide variety of concepts and variables contributing to risk, vulnerability, and resiliency among youth, it also focuses specifically on risk factors associated with AIDS, schizophrenia, eating disorders, depression, and attentional problems.

Chapter 26

American Nurses Association. 1994. *Psychiatric Mental Health Nursing Psychopharmacology Project.* Washington, DC: American Nurses Publishing.

This report from the task force on psychopharmacology reviews the current place of psychopharmacology in psychiatric nursing and sets the course for the future state of the art.

Gilman, S., & Newman, S. W. 1992. *Clinical neuroanatomy and neurophysiology,* 8th ed. Philadelphia: Davis.

This text provides a brief, but careful survey of brain anatomy and physiology. The text is supported by drawings of brain anatomy and diagrams that schematically represent brain function.

King, R. A., & Nosphitz, J. D. 1991. *Pathways of growth: Essentials of child psychiatry,* vol. 2—*Psychopathology.* New York: Wiley.

This volume, which deals with deviations from normal development, presents thoughtfully written chapters on psychiatric disorders of childhood.

Pennington, B. F. 1991. *Diagnosing learning disorders: A neuropsychological framework.* New York: Guilford Press.
A thorough review of current thinking on learning disabilities, it contains both theoretical and practical information.
Szatmari, P., Offord, D. R., & Boyle, M. H. 1989. Ontario Child Health Study: Prevalence of attention deficit disorder with hyperactivity. *Journal of Child Psychology and Psychiatry* 30: 219–30.
This is one of several published reports on a large epidemiologic study of psychiatric disorders in children and adolescents. Using careful sampling techniques, these investigators evaluated not only the frequency of psychiatric disorders in children and adolescents, but also the psychosocial correlates of these disorders and predictors of mental service use.

Chapter 27

Barbee, J. G., & McLaulin, J. B. 1990. Anxiety disorders: Diagnosis and pharmacotherapy in the elderly. *Psychiatric Annals* 29: 439–45.
The authors discuss clinical manifestations of anxiety disorders in the elderly and the treatment of these disorders with psychotherapy or pharmacotherapy.The authors take the position that the clinician must examine the client's nonspecific complaints in relation to presenting symptoms before administering medication. The pharmacologic approach recommended is a short-term course of anxiolytics, ideally benzodiazepines or buspirone.
Barresi, D. M., & Stull, D. E., eds. 1993. *Ethnic elderly and long-term care.* New York: Springer.
The authors include experts from a variety of academic disciplines, practitioners, planners, and policymakers. This book is organized into six sections that explore basic issues related to ethnicity in long-term care, caregiver issues in home-based long-term care, self-care practices, institutions that currently provide care and services in ethnically oriented settings, and planning, policy, and practice issues.
Cohen, G. D. 1990. Prevalence of psychiatric problems in older adults. *Psychiatric Annals* 20: 433–38.
This article assesses the impact of psychiatric problems in the over-65 population.. The author explores controversies over past and present clinical practice and research findings related to psychiatric problems of older adults, including depression, schizophrenia, Alzheimer's disease, suicide, other mental health problems, and the interaction between mental and physical health factors.
Gomez, G. E., & Gomez, E. A. 1990. The special concerns of neuroleptic use in the elderly. *Journal of Psychosocial Nursing and Mental Health Services* 23(1): 6–14.
This article is a comprehensive discussion of the use of neuroleptics in treating psychiatric disorders in the elderly. The authors conclude that elderly clients are prone to physiologic and psychological distress and are at risk when psychotropic interventions are used.
Roe, D. A. 1985. Therapeutic effects of drug-nutrient interactions in the elderly. *Journal of the American Dietetic Association* 85(2): 174–75, 181.
This article discusses the effects of food, specific nutrients in food, dietary fiber, and enteral feeding on the absorption of medications in the elderly. Also addressed is nutrient depletion as an adverse drug reaction.
Watanabe, M., & Davis, J. M. 1990. Overview: Pharmacotherapeutic considerations in the elderly psychiatric patient. *Psychiatric Annals* 20: 423–32.
This article discusses what clinicians need to know about pharmacotherapeutics to diagnose and treat psychiatric disorders effectively. Guidelines are presented on managing the risks of overdosing and toxicity problems in elderly psychiatric patients.

Chapter 28

Baker, S. G. 1994. Gender, ethnicity, and homelessness: Accounting for demographic diversity on the streets. *American Behavioral Scientist* 37(4): 476–504.
The author argues that it is the very heterogeneity of the homeless population in the United States that has stymied scholars and policymakers in their attempts to develop a comprehensive strategy for resolving the problem of homelessness. She cites recent research that high-

lights several interesting contrasts in the incidence of homelessness and in how homelessness is experienced by persons of different sexes and races.
Harris, S. N., Mowbray, C. T., & Solarz, A. 1994. Physical health, mental health, and substance abuse problems of shelter users. *Health and Social Work* 19(1): 37–45.
Working on the assumption that psychiatric problems, substance abuse, and physical health problems are all strongly interrelated for homeless persons, the authors thoroughly examines these factors among shelter users in Detroit.
Caton, C. L. M., Shrout, P. E., Eagle, P. F., et al. 1994. Risk factors for homelessness among schizophrenic men: A case-control study. *American Journal of Public Health* 84(2): 265–270.
The authors explore three areas of risk factors in a comparison of homeless and never-homeless schizophrenic men: severity of mental illness, family background, and prior use of mental health services.
Mowbray, C. T., Cohen, E., Harris, S., et al. 1992. Serving the homeless mentally ill: Mental health linkage. *Journal of Community Psychology,* 20: 215–27.
The authors argue that the services used to help the mentally ill must help the patient bridge the gap between a state of hopelessness and access to a future in which they can contribute to society as fully functioning members. The authors describe three demonstration project sites and how they met, or failed to meet, the expectations of the clientele served.

Chapter 29

Alcoholics Anonymous World Services, Inc. 1976. *Alcoholics Anonymous.* New York: Author.
Since 1939, this publication has been the blueprint for AA's recovery program. In addition to describing the program and how it works, the book contains first-person accounts by a number of people who have recovered from alcoholism.
Evans, K., & Sullivan, J. M. 1990. *Dual diagnosis: Counseling the mentally ill substance abuser.* New York: Guilford Press.
This is a practical and well-written handbook for health care personnel interested in understanding dual diagnosis. It offers suggestions for treatment planning.
Lowinson, J. H., Ruiz, P., Millman, R. B., & Langrod, J. G. 1992. *Substance abuse: A comprehensive textbook,* pp. 70–99. Baltimore: Williams & Wilkins.
This excellent reference describes numerous methods of treatment for substance abuse. The book includes a thorough discussion of the neurobiology of each abusable substance, and it explores historical, cultural, and policy issues in treatment.

Chapter 30

Burke, P. 1991. Depression in pediatric illness [Review]. *Behavior Modification* 15(4): 486–500.
In this discussion of depression as a complication of pediatric illness, the author reviews issues of assessment and diagnosis.
Gracely, R. H. 1995. Hypnosis and hierarchical pain control systems. *Pain* 60(1): 1–2.
This article describes the role and efficacy of hypnosis in pain amelioration and control.
Purcell, T. B. 1991. The somatic patient. *Emergency Medicine Clinics of North America* 9(1): 137–59.
The author describes methods of assessment to determine somatoform disorders.
Stout, S. C., & Nemeroff, C. B. 1994. Stress and psychiatric disorders. *Seminars in the Neurosciences* 6: 271–80.
This article explores the connection between the neurologic and immune systems and chronic stress and the resulting pathophysiologic feedback loop.
Turk, D. C., Brody, M. C., & Okifuji, E. A. 1994. Physicians' attitudes and practices regarding the long-term prescribing of opioids for non-cancer pain. *Pain* 59(2): 201–8.
Physicians' misplaced concern about drug dependence on opioids used in treating pain is the topic of this article.
Turk, D. C., & Melzack, R. 1992. The measurement of pain and the assessment of people experiencing pain. In D. C. Turk & R. Melzack, eds. *Handbook of pain assessment,* pp. 3–14. New York: Guilford.
This chapter offers a detailed presentation on and discussion of pain assessment and intervention.

Chapter 31

Teasdale, K. 1995. Theoretical and practical considerations on the use of reassurance in the nursing management of anxious patients. *Journal of Advanced Nursing* 22(1): 79–88.

This article analyzes the concept of reassurance in health care. The author argues that reassurance entails giving information and predicting a safe outcome. A survey concludes that reassuring strategies are indicated for patients whose fears are judged to be unrealistic or excessive.

Benham, E. 1995. Coping strategies: A psychoeducational approach to post-traumatic symptomatology. *Journal of Psychosocial Nursing and Mental Health Services* 33(6): 30–35, 40–41.

Survivors of extensive childhood abuse frequently present complicated clinical dilemmas in the inpatient setting; they experience complex post-traumatic and dissociative symptomatology, such as flashbacks and other reexperiencing phenomena, as well as intense affects and self-destructive impulses. Such patients seek recommendations on how to manage their post-traumatic symptoms, as well as how to tolerate intense affects and maintain safety. Coping strategies, which the patients learn to formulate, help clients stall impulsivity and dissociative episodes through the use of healthy diversions, grounding techniques, and support networks.

Liveley, S., Friedrich, R., & Buckwalter, K. 1995. Sibling perception of schizophrenia: Impact on relationships, roles, and health. *Issues in Mental Health Nursing* 16(3) 225–38.

The impact of schizophrenia on 30 adult siblings of patients with schizophrenia was examined. Siblings' perceptions of its impact on roles, relationships, and health were investigated, revealing that patients with schizophrenia experience changes in all relationships but especially those with their siblings. The more severe the schizophrenia, the greater the impact on the sibling.

Smith, B., Mitchell, A., Bruno, A., & Constantino, R. 1995. Exploring widows' experiences after the suicide of their spouse. *Journal of Psychosocial Nursing and Mental Health Services* 33(5): 10–15, 42–43.

The widows of spouses who commit suicide must cope with issues related to depression, anger, blame, guilt, and the stigma associated with suicide. Thus, recovery from this type of loss is different for the survivors than recovery from other types of crises. The predominant need of widows and widowers of suicide victims is to talk in an environment of acceptance and understanding, which can only be provided by other people who have had the same kind of experience.

Chapter 32

Lerner, H. 1986. *The dance of anger: A woman's guide to changing the patterns of intimate relationships.* New York: Harper & Row.

The author explores women's experience of anger and the influence of anger on their personal relationships, drawing from clinical experiences and research to highlight how anger can hinder people from making changes in relationships. Specific strategies are provided for making behavior changes and improving self-esteem.

Miedzan, M. 1991. *Boys will be boys: Breaking the link between masculinity and violence.* Toronto: Doubleday.

The author explores the values of the American culture that promote and maintain the role of men as tough, dominant, and competitive and as people who deny empathy. After exploring the values and assumptions, she addresses ways of parenting and socializing male children with less emphasis on values and assumptions that promote violence.

Morrison, E. F. 1993. Toward a better understanding of violence in psychiatric settings: Debunking the myths. *Archives of Psychiatric Nursing* 7(6): 328–35.

The author invites the reader to reconsider the view that violence in psychiatric settings is different from violence in other settings. Because of five myths or assumptions held by many health care professionals, health care professionals sometimes do not institute consequences after a violent incident, fail to set clear behavioral expectations, or blame the victim or health care staff for violent episodes. Morrison concludes by postulating that violence in psychiatric settings is similar to violence in any part of society and is best viewed as a social problem, not a medical or psychological one.

Maier, G. 1996. Managing threatening behavior. The role of talk down and talk up. *Journal of Psychosocial Nursing* 34(6): 25–30.

This article discusses hot and cold threats of persons with Axis I and Axis II disorders. Understanding these general diagnostic differences can help the nurse plan safe management approaches.

Chapter 33

Campbell, J., & Humphreys, J. 1993. *Nursing care of survivors of family violence,* pp. 69–104. St. Louis: Mosby.
An excellent reference for nurses, this book provides comprehensive coverage of all forms of abuse and the nursing care of survivors of abuse.
Dutton, D. G. 1995. *The domestic assault of women.* Vancouver, British Columbia, Canada: UBC Press.
This book, which is more appropriate for professionals than most lay readers, covers all aspects of domestic assault and reviews pertinent research. The book includes an in-depth discussion of traumatic bonding.
Herman, J. L. 1992. *Trauma and recovery.* New York: Basic Books.
This book covers PTSD and trauma, its consequences, and the process of recovery in depth. The book is more appropriate for professionals than most lay readers.
NiCarthy, G. 1986. *Getting free: You can end abuse and take back your life.* Seattle: Seal Press.
This easy-to-read book is directed to survivors of abuse and is intended to help them understand violent relationships and ways to end violence.
NiCarthy, G. 1987. *The ones who got away: Women who left abusive partners.* Seattle, Wash: Seal Press.
This book presents stories of abused women who were able to end their violent relationships. It is excellent for readers who want first-hand accounts of what it means to be entrapped in a violent relationship.
Walker, L. 1979. *The battered women.* New York: Harper & Row.
This classic work was one of the first comprehensive books on the topic of domestic violence. It describes the cycle of violence. Appropriate for lay persons and professionals, the book is easy to read.

Chapter 34

Juon, H. S. & Ensminger, M. E. 1997. Child, adolescent, and young adult predictors of suicidal behaviors: A prospective study of African Americans. *Journal of Child Psychology and Psychiatry* 38(5): 553–63.
This study examined the lifetime prevalence of suicidal behaviors and their relation to social integration, depression, and aggression/substance use in a cohort of African Americans followed prospectively from first grade to age 32. The results suggest that social integration, depression, and aggression/drug use are important risk factors for suicidal behaviors in this population.
Brent, D. A. 1997. The aftercare of adolescents with deliberate self harm. *Journal of Child Psychology and Psychiatry* 38(3): 277–86.
The evaluation and aftercare of the adolescent suicide attempter is described. Important elements of treatment include obtaining a no-suicide contract, addressing potential sources of noncompliance, determining proper intensity of treatment, provision of family psychoeducation addressing ongoing family difficulties, treatment of co-occurring psychopathology, and remediation of social skills and problem-solving deficits.
John, D. S. 1996. The suicidal patient: Identifying, evaluating, and intervening. *Home Care Provider* 1(5): 246–53.
Patients who demonstrate self wound behavior require behavioral, pharmacological, and psychotherapeutic interventions to meet their highly complex needs. Nurses caring for these patients will experience frustration related to the safety needs of the patients and guilt whenever an injury occurs.
Egan, M. P., Rivera, S. G., Robillard, R. R., & Hanson, A. 1997. The no-suicide contract: Helpful or harmful? *Journal of Psychosocial Nursing* 35(3): 31–33.
Contracting for safety (CFS) has become an integral part of nursing practice. The author argues that CFS can, in some instances, be helpful in establishing a therapeutic relationship or aiding in assessment, but never should be the sole basis for determining a patient's lethality.
Tapp, A. 1997. Supervision of psychiatric patients. *Canadian Nurse* 93(3): 47–48.

This article addresses the amount of supervision or intervention required to protect a patient from self harm or from injuring others from a legal and health care perspective.
Samuelsson, M., Asberg, M., & Gustavsson, J. P. 1997. Attitudes of psychiatric nursing personnel towards patients who have attempted suicide. *Acta Psychiatric Scananavia* 95(#): 222–30.
The aim of this study was to examine the attitudes towards suicidal patients of a group of psychiatric nursing personnel and to establish a baseline of attitudinal measures against which the effects of a subsequent educational program can be assessed. Differences between personnel working in different settings were found.
Viens, C. 1997. Developing expertise in the rural milieu. *Canadian Nurse* 93(2): 39–42.
This article explores the health of the farming family, identifying isolation, stress, psychological distress, violence, drug and alcohol abuse, suicide, and the health risks of farming itself. The farming family is largely misunderstood and presents a sizable challenge to researchers and health care providers.

Chapter 35

Blair, T., & Dauner, A. 1993. Neuroleptic malignant syndrome: Liability in nursing practice. *Journal of Psychosocial Nursing* 31(2): 5–12.
The authors provide a timely and significant discussion of the need for nurses to become familiar with NMS. They review the malpractice case of Reyes v Houston International Hospital, which involved a nearly fatal case of NMS, and emphasize the need for nurses to remain aware of the legal ramifications of administering medications in a psychiatric setting.
Caroff, S., & Mann, S. 1993. Neuroleptic malignant syndrome. *Medical Clinics of North America* 77(1): 185–202.
A thorough review of the current state of research on NMS, including risk factors, clinical course, differential diagnosis, and treatment, this article is recommended for nurses who need a comprehensive reference on NMS or wish to explore the topic in depth.
Hyman, S. 1994. Acute drug overdose. In S. Hyman & G. Tesar, ed. *Manual of psychiatric emergencies,* pp. 304–22. Boston: Little, Brown.
This chapter explains the general principles of emergency treatment of drug overdoses. It covers specific issues that arise in overdoses of psychiatric drugs. Toxic effects of acute overdoses of sedative-hypnotics, tricyclic and other cyclic antidepressants, lithium, MAOIs, and neuroleptic drugs are listed in an easy-to-use reference format.
Snider, K., & Boyd, M. 1991. When they drink too much: Nursing interventions for patients with disordered water balance. *Journal of Psychosocial Nursing* 29(7): 10–16.
The authors present a general overview of disordered water balance and further categorize this disorder into three levels of severity: mild, moderate, and severe. A table included in the article provides a useful description of the physiologic, behavioral, and cognitive changes associated with each of these three levels. Appropriate nursing care diagnoses and interventions for each level of disordered water balance are thoroughly discussed.
Riggs, A., Dyksen, M., Kim, S., & Opsahl, J. 1991. A review of disorders of water homeostasis in psychiatric patients. *Psychosomatics* 32(2): 133–48.
This article discusses in depth the mechanisms of thirst, vasopressin release, and inappropriate secretion of antidiuretic hormone. In addition, the article presents a historical review of water imbalance disorders and a comprehensive critique of current research on their etiology and treatment.

Answer Section

1 ▪ *The changing perception of mental health*

Matching

1. c 2. e 3. a 4. d 5. b

Labeling

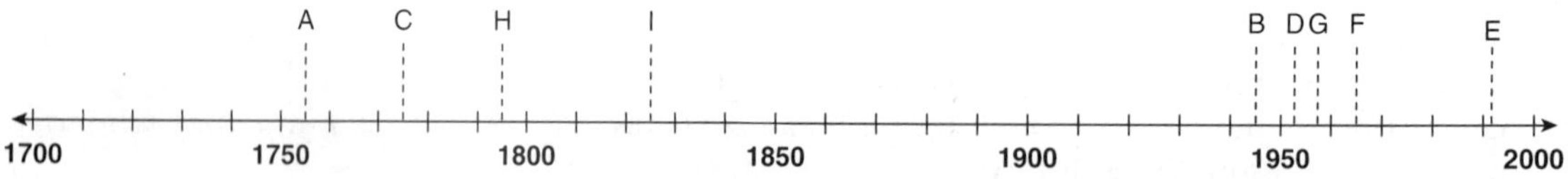

Multiple choice

1. c 2. a 3. b 4. d 5. c

2 ▪ *Cultural issues related to mental health care*

Word find

```
N O T E R O N K S Y X Z I M A S I T E
I C E D T G I N M E Y T I D N I E Y G
O R S Y M P H O C B G I A E G P O U R
N I S A O Z M B U I L R D R N T L C E
P A J K H A T R L A S P E N E G I M A
E L I T N I U G T R O N S G R D K P O
A Y W E X M N A U U Y S I T A U T B M
Z P Z C G A O T R A J N S R C T H O A
I D P U R G I G A T B O P N R T I A H
M J H D O A T O L R I I E O N M A O L
G R O A U P A C C U L T U R A T I O N
A C C U P A Z N O I T A J E R P B A K
T U B I D W I W M E A R N B E D O H J
S T E R E O T Y P I N G M R I O H O M
E L M A N S A M E L Z E U S T Y P I E
G R O D S V M K T X M T C U L T O C F
R E H B I O G I E Q L N I A C F M T S
A U G C T A I V N U J I U K I O O I T
G S D S Y M T E C I D U J E R P H O L
E M A N L I S T E R E O T P P Y I N G
```

Fill in the blanks

1. Acculturation
2. Stigmatization
3. Prejudice; dislocation and change; cultural isolation and absence of social support; and identity localization.
4. Family
5. Supernatural intervention or evil or vengeful spirits
6. Learning and age
7. Decreased
8. Outbreak of AIDS
9. Internalize, negative
10. Biologic
11. The decade of the brain
12. Biases and prejudice

Multiple choice

1. b 2. c 3. c 4. a 5. b 6. d 7. a

3 ▪ *The mental health-mental illness continuum and decision making*

Short answer

1. Ability to function
2. Return of symptoms, functional ability, distress experienced, and cultural and societal norms
3. Severe and persistent mental illness
4. Descriptive, analytic, and experimental
5. Establishing of specific criteria for diagnosis
6. ICD 10 and DSM IV
7. Inquisitive, well informed, trustful of reason, open minded, flexible, fair in evaluation, honest in facing personal biases, careful in judgements, and willing to reconsider previous judgements.
8. To provide a guide for clinical practice
9. Reduce incidence(primary prevention); lower prevalence (secondary prevention); and lower the rate of residual disability (tertiary prevention)
10. Maintenance interventions

Word unscramble

1. Algorithms
2. Epidemiology
3. Risk factors
4. Dimensional diagnoses
5. Axes
6. Prevalence
7. Deductive approach

Multiple choice

1. b 2. a 3. c 4. a 5. d 6. b 7. d 8. c

4 ▪ *Consumer issues and treatment ethics*

Matching

1. d 2. a 3. f 4. g 5. i 6. h 7. b 8. j 9. e 10. c

Sentence correction

1. The patient's right to refuse treatment is based on self determination.
2. True
3. Most states provide for emergency short term hospitalization of 48 to 92 hours.
4. Guilty by mentally ill individuals are remanded to correctional system. Not guilty by reason of insanity individuals are committed to the mental health system.
5. The American Public Health Association is an example of an external advocacy system.
6. True
7. A statistical ethical model bases treatment decisions on previous statistics and results; an individual ethical model bases treatment decisions on the individual's unique situation.
8. True
9. True
10. True

Multiple choice

1. c 2. b 3. a 4. d 5. d 6. b

5 ▪ *The shaping of contemporary psychiatric nursing practice*

Fill in the blanks

1. Moral Treatment
2. McLean Asylum training school
3. Body and soul
4. Nursing Mental Disorders
5. Therapeutic relationship
6. Professional standards
7. Baccalaureate
8. American Psychiatric Nurses Association (APNA)
9. Initiation, stabilization, maintenance, and discontinuation and follow up
10. Patterns; processes

Labeling

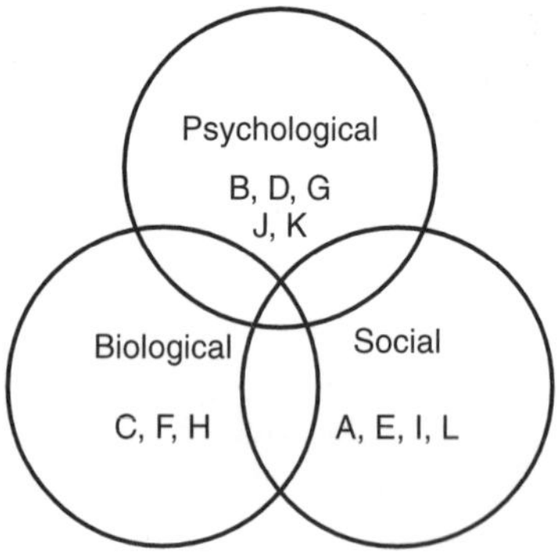

Multiple choice

1. b 2. d 3. c 4. a 5. c 6. b 7. d 8. a 9. c

6 ▪ *Theoretical basis of psychiatric nursing*

Matching

1. l 2. h 3. i 4. m 5. b 6. g 7. n 8. f 9. d 10. e 11. o 12. a 13. j 14. c 15. k

Word find

L	I	F	E	S	P	A	C	E	E	F	I	F	T	E
T	Y	G	R	I	D	N	S	L	N	I	F	R	C	S
P	L	S	Y	S	O	X	O	E	M	R	U	S	M	N
M	I	C	H	E	M	R	C	R	I	S	U	S	A	E
N	C	P	T	N	G	T	I	M	T	R	S	E	E	F
A	M	A	A	E	I	Y	A	O	E	G	G	N	R	D
C	A	K	P	G	N	I	L	E	D	O	M	S	A	M
C	F	A	M	I	L	Y	D	Y	N	A	M	I	C	S
O	N	X	E	P	T	O	I	E	N	Y	D	P	F	I
M	O	D	L	E	U	T	S	T	N	E	C	E	L	U
M	L	O	I	B	J	R	T	R	C	I	E	R	E	R
O	A	X	W	V	O	S	A	O	J	L	A	G	S	T
D	N	E	H	I	R	P	N	P	M	D	N	L	O	L
A	E	P	E	S	P	E	C	N	G	I	R	I	T	A
T	R	E	T	O	D	L	E	M	P	U	W	K	C	N
I	O	C	R	A	M	O	L	A	F	A	B	E	S	D
O	J	T	P	R	A	T	H	I	E	O	N	L	I	C
N	O	I	T	C	A	S	N	A	R	T	Z	A	T	A

Short answer

1. Genetic vulnerability predisposes a person to a disorder; when combined with environmental stressors, the abnormal behavior occurs
2. Id, ego, and superego
3. Sense of inferiority as the motivating force in human life; person from birth continually striving to overcome it
4. Situation neuroses: from anxiety of a single conflict; character neuroses: from a basic anxiety and hostility resulting from a lack of love and affection in childhood
5. According to Sullivan, interpersonal relationships, not sexual or aggressive instinctual drives central for personality development; anxiety defined differently to include all types of emotional suffering
6. Empathy and positive regard
7. Classical view—undesirable conscious emotional reaction to a patient that reflects analyst's unresolved conflict; totalistic view—all the therapist's feelings, and attitudes toward the patient
8. a. Rationalization
   b. Displacement
   c. Projection
   d. Reaction formation
   e. Repression
   f. Suppression
   g. Acting out
9. Principle of frequency and recency
10. Intelligence viewed as an adaptation to environment that grows from an organized structure becoming differentiated over time; linked to mental embryology

11. Impact on the parent's or family members' patterns and unresolved conflicts or losses of the family of origin
12. Orientation, working, and termination
13. Rapport
14. To promote adaptation with adaptive responses
15. Emphasis on promoting independence and self care because psychiatric disorders often manifested as difficulties conducting ordinary self care activities or developing independent thinking skills

Multiple choice

1. b 2. a 3. d 4. b 5. c 6. d 7. d 8. a 9. c 10. b

7 ▪ *The biologic foundations of psychiatric nursing*

Labeling

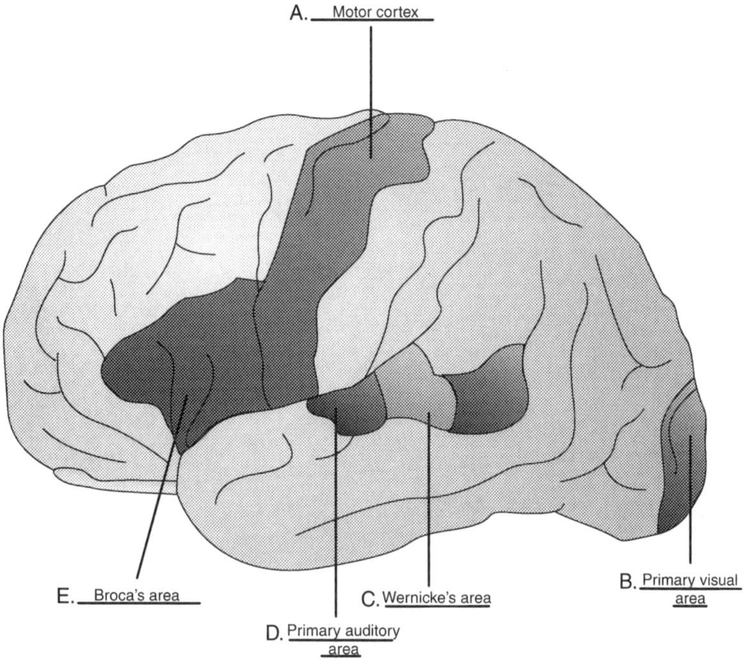

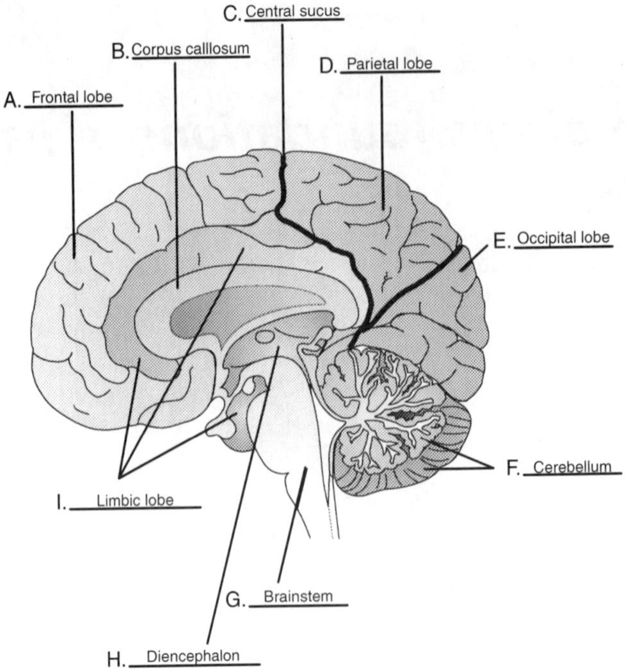
C. Central sucus
B. Corpus calllosum
D. Parietal lobe
A. Frontal lobe
E. Occipital lobe
F. Cerebellum
I. Limbic lobe
G. Brainstem
H. Diencephalon

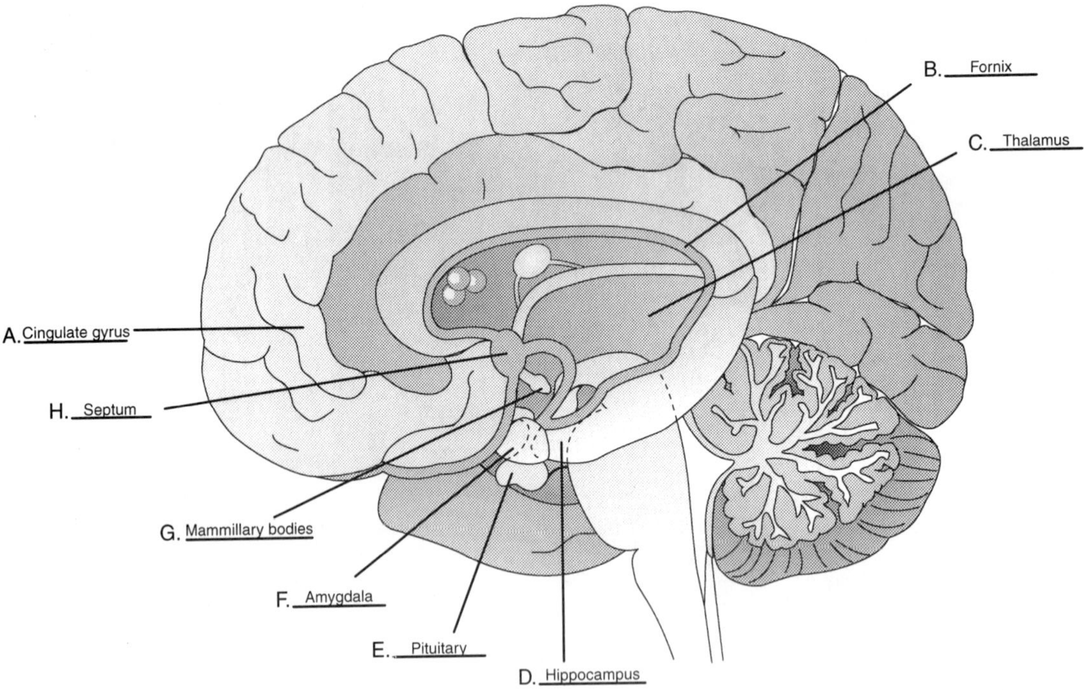
B. Fornix
C. Thalamus
A. Cingulate gyrus
H. Septum
G. Mammillary bodies
F. Amygdala
E. Pituitary
D. Hippocampus

Fill in the blanks

1. Cerebrospinal fluid; choroid plexus
2. Cytoarchitecture
3. Plasticity
4. Sulci; fissures
5. Central sulcus
6. Hippocampus
7. Midbrain, pons, and medulla
8. Raphe system
9. Axon; dendrites
10. Calcium
11. Acetylcholine
12. Zeitgebers
13. Challenge test
14. Alpha; beta; theta or delta
15. a. Parasympathetic
    b. Sympathetic
    c. Sympathetic
    d. Parasympathetic
    e. Sympathetic
    f. Parasympathetic
    g. Sympathetic

Multiple choice

1. b 2. a 3. d 4. b 5. c 6. a 7. d 8. b 9. c 10. a

8 ▪ *The basics of biologic treatments*

Labeling

1. A. Acetylcholine
   B. Dopamine
   C. Norepinephrine
   D. Serotonin

2. a. B (Dopamine)
   b. A and C (Acetylcholine and Norepinephrine)
   c. C and D (Norepinephrine and Serotonin)
   d. C (Norepinephrine)
   e. D (Serotonin)
   f. B (Dopamine)
   g. A and C (Acetylcholine and Norepinephrine)
   h. A (Acetylcholine)
   i. C (Norepinephrine)

Crossword puzzle

															1 P		
															H		
2 P	S	Y	C	H	O	P	H	A	3 R	M	4 A	C	O	L	O	G	Y
H									E		G				T		
A									C		O				O		
R									E		N				T		
M									P		I				H		
5 A	N	T	6 A	G	O	N	I	S	T		S				E		
C			K						O		7 T	A	P	E	R		
O			A						R						A		
8 D	Y	S	T	O	N	I	A			9 A					P		
Y			H					10 E	F	F	I	C	A	C	Y		
N			I							F							
A			S		11 D	I	S	T	R	I	B	U	T	I	O	N	
M			I							N							
I			A				12 T	O	X	I	C	I	T	Y			
C										T							
13 S	E	L	E	C	T	I	V	I	T	Y							

Multiple choice

1. b 2. a 3. d 4. c 5. c 6. b 7. b 8. a 9. c 10. b 11. d 12. d 13. a 14. c 15. b

9 ▪ *Communication and the therapeutic relationship*

Word unscramble

1. Nonverbal communication
2. Symbolism
3. Resolution
4. Boundaries
5. Rapport
6. Reflection
7. Self awareness
8. Verbal contract
9. Empathy
10. Themes

Multiple choice

1. c 2. b 3. d 4. b 5. a 6. c 7. a 8. d 9. b 10. d

10 ▪ *The assessment process*

Crossword puzzle

											1 A	F	F	E	C	T
			2 I								S					
			N								S					
			3 S	E	L	F	4 E	S	T	E	E	M				
			I				U				S					
5 J	U	D	G	M	E	N	T				S					
			H				H				M					
			T				Y			6 R	E	C	A	L	L	
		7 M					M				N					
	8 C	O	G	N	I	T	I	O	N		T					
		O					C									
		D														

Fill in the blanks

1. Ongoing
2. Patient interview
3. Own sexuality
4. Mental status exam
5. Affect
6. Mini Mental state exam
7. Body image, self-esteem, and personal identity

Multiple choice

1. c 2. b 3. a 4. b 5. d 6. a 7. b 8. c 9. d

11 ▪ *Diagnosis and outcomes development*

Short answer

1. Objective and subjective signs and symptoms of the nursing assessment
2. Outcomes
3. Planning
4. Outcome criteria
5. Continuous quality improvement (CQI)
6. Subject, verb, circumstances, and standard of performance
7. Pathophysiologic, maturational, situational, and treatment related

Word find

```
T C T I V E O S T U O C
U R O U T C U O D S M E
O I A R T D T M E D E C
E T G E I E C M F O L N
V E E H N F O T I I N A
I R N A I C M O N M U M
T S S B T I E I I A R R
A E R U I N C P N I S O
G M O L A A R R G N I F
E O T I L G I A C C N R
N C C P O D T C H S G E
I T A T U I E T A T D P
N T F A T S R I R N I F
H A D T C C I C A A A O
A R E I O H A A C E G D
M I T O M R T I T M N R
U A A N E G N L E E O A
H H L P S I G A R T S D
B K E M L S T Y I L I N
E T R C F S C T S A S A
F O N T A R L O T T T T
O P A H T I S R I S C S
C H A R A C T E C R I S
```

Multiple choice

1. b 2. d 3. c 4. b 5. b 6. b 7. c

12 ▪ *Biopsychosocial interventions*

Matching

1. g 2. i 3. f 4. h 5. d 6. a 7. j 8. c 9. b 10. e

Labeling

Basic Physiologic B, E	Complex Physiologic D, F, L
Behavioral A, I	Safety C, K
Family F, J	Health System G, H

Fill in the blanks

1. Nurse-patient relationship
2. Distraction
3. Calmness, objectivity
4. Catharsis, problem solving, insight
5. Psychoeducation
6. Closed
7. 8 to 10, more than 10
8. Inclusion, control, and affection
9. Group themes
10. Validation

Multiple choice

1. b 2. c 3. d 4. a 5. c 6. c 7. a 8. b

13 ▪ *Nursing practice within the continuum of care*

Word find

```
V I C T Y C M A N A G E K A R E D L N T
M O D L E O L S T A B I L I Z A T I O N
S T O U R N C U N T R T R E E T M O I E
V A Y Z L T R Y B Q A R S U T O E N T M
X C H G W I U G P H C O N P I R T M A E
O X F T B N X R S Z O W E V A C N O R G
T E I T N U T A Y I R U T I C R O N G A
D D W S I U V E C H A M S I T E C T E N
N U V E L M O R E L A P S E U T A I T A
F L M N O O E L E R E F A L M Z Y V N M
L A R R E F E R I F H O I O N O B E I E
A J K S S C D T O X I C A T P S D D E S
G N I N N A L P E G R A H C S I D E R A
R P A Q R R X O M L A S P R E R A L L C
A R F O S E T R E R A C K O F T I A N N
T O X I F I C A T I O N D E R E S I D E
```

Short answer

1. In 1960, by J. F. Kennedy with the need for more community services
2. Through voluntary admission or involuntary commitment
3. Hospitalization or a minimum of 90 days but less than 120 days
4. Short-term treatment
5. Control of precipitating symptoms with medications, behavioral interventions, and coordination with other agencies for aftercare
6. Increase patient's ability to function within the home and decrease hospitalizations
7. Moral/spiritual foundation, assessment, relationship building, medication issues, patient education/psychotherapeutic intervention and case management
8. Personal care homes, board and care homes, therapeutic foster care, and supervised apartments
9. Reintegration of people back into the community through work, educational, and social avenues
10. Medications, ADLs, mental health aftercare, residence, physical health care follow-up and special education, financial or other need.

Multiple choice

1. b 2. a 3. b 4. c 5. a 6. d 7. d 8. d

14 ▪ *Schizophrenia*

Matching

1. e 2. g 3. i 4. a 5. j 6. b 7. c 8. d 9. h 10. f

Short answer

1. a. Positive; b. Negative; c. Positive; d. Negative; e. Positive; f. Positive; g. Positive; h. Negative
2. a. Phase II; b. Phase I; c. Phase III; d. Phase III; e. Phase II
3. Men
4. Depression and substance abuse
5. Enlarged lateral ventricle, enlarged 3rd ventricle, and enlarged sulci
6. Nigrostriatal dopaminergic tract
7. Elevated temperature greater than 99°F with no apparent cause
8. Initiation, stabilization, and maintenance
9. Catatonic state and depression not treatable by other means
10. Auditory hallucinations

Multiple choice

1. c 2. b 3. a 4. d 5. b 6. a 7. a 8. b 9. c 10. d 11. c 12. d

15 ▪ *Schizoaffective, delusional, and other psychotic disorders*

Word unscramble

1. Psychosis
2. Thymoleptic
3. Delusions
4. Erotomania
5. Misidentification

Fill in the blanks

1. Bipolar
2. Smaller, asymmetry
3. Dopamine pathway
4. Panic attacks
5. Valproate
6. Self harm
7. High
8. Tactile, somatic or olfactory
9. Bodily function
10. Middle to late adulthood

Multiple choice

1. b 2. c 3. a 4. a 5. d 6. b 7. c

16 ▪ *Mood disorders*

Labeling

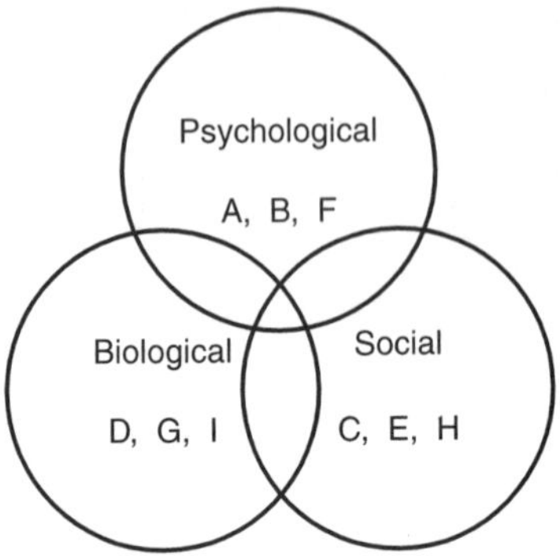

Tricyclic	*SSRI*	*MAOIs*	*Other atypical*
B, D	A, E	C, G	F, H

Word find

E	L	E	C	T	D	L	R	O	C	O	N	V	U	E	L	S	I
E	U	P	H	O	T	A	S	E	R	O	T	O	N	L	I	N	G
R	A	L	O	P	I	B	P	Y	L	A	B	I	L	E	T	Y	N
A	R	M	R	D	Y	I	A	A	N	R	E	H	T	V	E	V	I
L	P	A	I	E	H	L	I	P	O	D	O	R	M	A	P	X	L
O	E	N	A	A	A	I	R	O	H	P	U	E	I	T	O	R	C
P	S	I	A	F	H	T	O	T	A	Y	G	R	X	E	L	D	Y
I	S	C	F	N	A	Y	H	R	I	L	I	N	O	D	A	I	C
N	I	E	T	I	E	X	P	A	N	S	I	V	E	M	O	O	D
U	C	P	H	A	S	E	S	O	A	I	P	E	D	O	M	S	I
T	O	I	E	P	O	Y	Y	P	M	Y	P	I	E	O	I	E	P
R	N	S	Y	R	A	P	D	I	O	A	C	D	R	D	S	O	A
D	Y	O	I	N	T	E	R	D	R	P	N	X	P	A	N	R	R
M	H	D	S	S	O	N	A	L	E	E	R	I	A	B	V	D	O
P	S	E	U	D	O	D	E	M	E	N	T	I	A	S	R	E	R

Multiple choice

1. c 2. d 3. b 4. a 5. d 6. c 7. d 8. a 9. b 10. a 11. c 12. b

17 ▪ *Anxiety and related disorders*

Crossword puzzle

											1 A	N	X	I	E	T	Y
2 P	A	N	I	3 C							G						
				4 O	B	S	E	S	S	I	O	N	S				
				M							R						5 C
				P							A						U
				U				6 I	M	I	P	R	A	M	I	N	E
				L							H						C
				S							O						A
				I							B						R
		7 C	L	O	M	I	P	R	A	M	I	N	E				D
				N							A						
				S													

Fill in the blanks

1. Overwhelming anxiety
2. a. affective; b. cognitive; c. physical; d. cognitive; e. behavioral; f. physical; g. behavioral
3. Fear of falling asleep
4. Women, men
5. Locus ceruleus
6. Anxiolytic and anxiogenic
7. Corticotropin releasing factor (CRF)
8. a. Psychodynamic theory; b. Psychoanalytic theory; c. Cognitive/behavioral (learning) theory
9. Anticholinergic
10. Exposure therapy
11. Overstimulation or repeated stimulation
12. Caffeine
13. Contamination
14. SSRIs
15. Identity, memory, and consciousness

Multiple choice

1. c 2. d 3. c 4. a 5. b 6. d 7. b 8. a 9. d 10. c 11. b 12. a 13. a 14. a

18 ▪ *Personality and impulse-control disorders*

Matching

1. k 2. f 3. l 4. j 5. b 6. i 7. g 8. c 9. a 10. e 11. h 12. d

Short answer

1. Correct the tendency to fulfill all the patient's needs by focusing on others to the exclusion of themselves
2. Parent overvaluation and overindulgence of child
3. Mistrust of others and desire to avoid relationships in which they are not in control or lose power
4. Increase the patient's ability to feel pleasure
5. Social skills training and environmental management
6. Negative comments and disapproval
7. Avoidant personality disorder
8. Low serotonin-norepinephrine levels
9. Increased tension immediately before pulling out the hair or when attempting to resist the behavior; sense of relief after hair is pulled out.
10. Winning, losing, desperation, and hopelessness

Multiple choice

1. a 2. c 3. d 4. b 5. c 6. a 7. d 8. c 9. b 10. d 11. a 12. b

19 ▪ *Somatoform and related disorders*

Word unscramble

1. Hypochondriasis
2. Somatization
3. Internalization
4. Psychosomatic
5. Malingering

Labeling

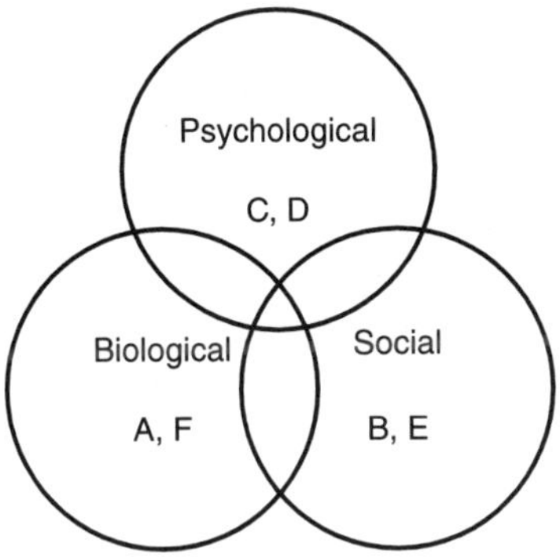

Multiple choice

1. b 2. c 3. d 4. c 5. a 6. b 7. b 8. a

20 · *Neuropsychiatric disorders*

Word find

T	A	M	U	I	R	I	L	E	D
A	I	S	O	N	G	A	B	A	A
E	T	M	M	E	M	P	O	I	I
S	N	I	X	U	D	R	S	A	S
A	E	N	A	R	Y	A	R	R	E
E	M	E	I	O	H	X	O	Y	N
S	E	U	P	P	A	I	P	O	I
I	D	R	A	S	S	A	T	R	K
D	U	O	C	Y	H	Y	A	H	Y
S	O	I	O	C	K	I	C	K	D
K	P	G	R	H	S	A	H	I	A
C	O	G	N	I	T	I	O	N	R
I	O	I	N	A	L	F	F	E	B
P	K	G	I	T	K	E	I	S	R
T	A	T	N	R	O	S	D	Y	A
D	E	M	E	Y	R	O	M	E	M

Matching

1. g 2. d 3. e 4. f 5. b 6. h 7. a 8. c

Multiple choice

1. a 2. c 3. b 4. d 5. d 6. b 7. a 8. c 9. b 10. a 11. d 12. d 13. a

21 ▪ *Eating disorders*

Fill in the blanks

1. Gender identity
2. Body image
3. Norepinephrine
4. Serotonin
5. Fluoxetine (Prozac)
6. Amenorrhea
7. Albumin
8. Benevolent ignorance
9. Binge purge
10. Bupropion

Crossword puzzle

1 T			2 N											
H			3 O	S	T	E	O	P	O	R	O	4 S	I	S
R			R									A		
O			5 E	N	M	E	S	H	M	E	N	T		
M			P									I		
6 B	U	L	I	M	I	A						E		
O			N									T		
C			E									Y		
Y			7 P	R	O	Z	A	C						
T			H											
O			R											
8 P	E	R	I	M	Y	O	9 L	Y	S	I	S			
E			N				A							
N			E				N							
I							U							
A							G							
							O							

Multiple choice

1. d 2. b 3. d 4. c 5. a 6. d 7. b 8. a 9. c 10. b

22 ▪ *Substance abuse disorders*

Labeling

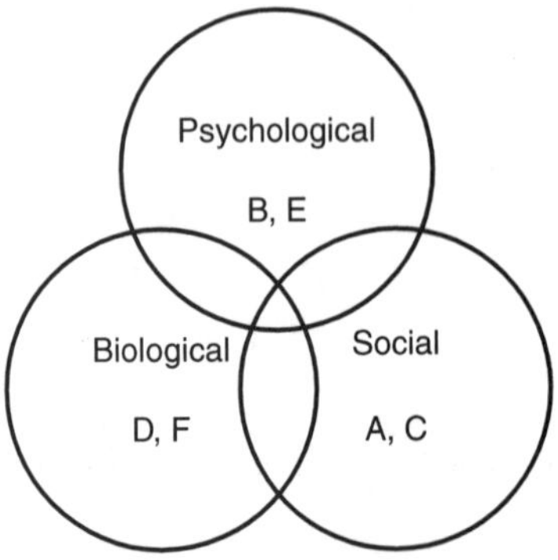

Matching

1. f 2. i 3. g 4. h 5. a 6. j 7. b 8. d 9. c 10. e

Multiple choice

1. c 2. b 3. a 4. d 5. b 6. c 7. d 8. c 9. b 10. a

23 ▪ *Sleep disorders*

Fill in the blanks

1. Circadian
2. Reticular activation system (RAS)
3. Sleep architecture
4. III and IV
5. 17 to 18 hours
6. Zeitgebers
7. Dyssomnias
8. Fall asleep or maintain sleep
9. Stimulus control
10. Daytime sleepiness, cataplexy, hypnagogic hallucinations, and sleep paralysis
11. Nocturnal enuresis
12. Melatonin
13. REM
14. Sleep walking

Multiple choice

1. c 2. b 3. d 4. a 5. b 6. c 7. a

24 ▪ *Sexual disorders*

Word unscramble

1. Fetishism
2. Paraphilias
3. Gender identity
4. Menopause
5. Dyspareunia
6. Orgasm
7. Excitement
8. Exhibitionism

Labeling

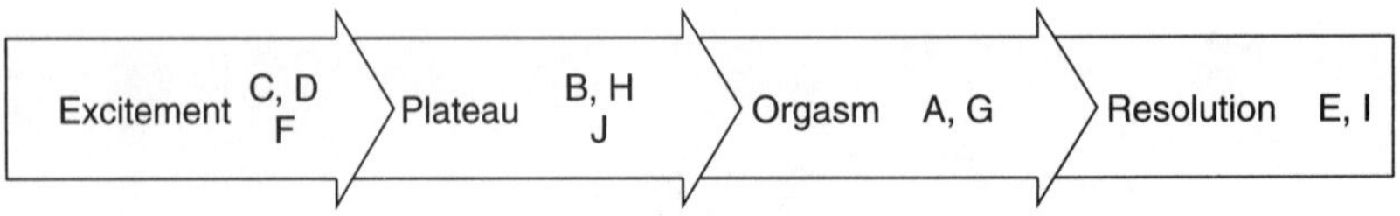

Multiple choice

1. d 2. c 3. a 4. b 5. c 6. d 7. a 8. b

25 ▪ *Mental health promotion with children and adolescents*

Matching

1. g 2. j 3. a 4. h 5. i 6. d 7. e 8. b 9. f 10. c

Labeling

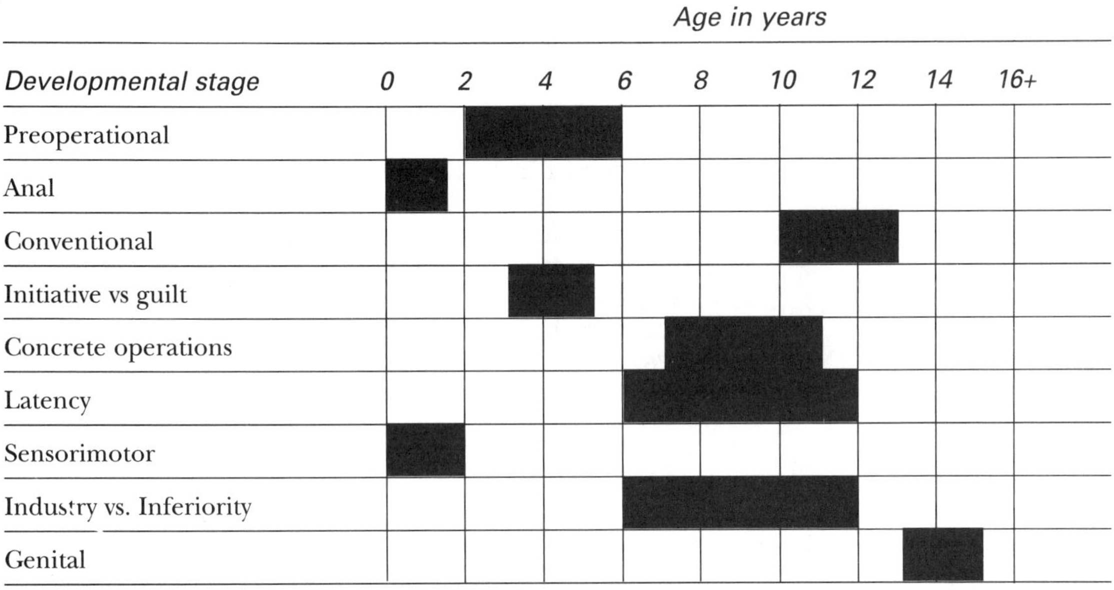

Multiple choice

1. c 2. b 3. a 4. d 5. b 6. d 7. b 8. c 9. a 10. d

26 ▪ *Care of children and adolescents with psychiatric disorders*

Word find

I	N	T	E	R	M	O	D	A	L	S	I	S	M	L	E
Y	C	O	N	D	U	C	T	D	I	S	O	R	D	E	R
T	D	E	V	E	L	O	Y	P	M	E	N	T	E	A	E
A	I	S	I	S	E	R	P	O	C	N	E	O	S	R	T
I	S	T	L	E	N	M	U	H	H	E	C	U	E	N	S
B	N	A	Z	L	O	S	N	B	Y	V	H	R	N	I	B
O	A	T	E	D	I	E	T	I	P	I	O	E	S	N	E
H	I	S	C	I	T	I	X	A	E	S	L	D	I	G	H
P	X	O	R	R	N	T	A	I	R	L	A	I	T	D	A
L	E	N	U	R	E	S	I	S	A	U	L	S	I	I	V
O	L	I	N	G	T	U	E	R	A	P	I	O	Z	S	P
O	S	M	E	N	T	A	D	U	C	M	A	R	A	O	R
H	Y	P	E	R	A	C	T	I	V	I	T	Y	T	R	O
C	D	A	T	T	E	I	N	O	T	I	V	T	I	D	D
S	N	O	I	T	S	T	T	E	R	U	O	T	O	E	E
O	I	T	A	M	C	I	N	U	M	M	O	C	N	R	R

Fill in the blanks

1. Mental retardation
2. Early age of onset and severe disturbance in social relatedness
3. Stereotypic behavior
4. Asperger's
5. Seizure
6. Milieu management
7. Phonological processing
8. Left; right
9. Education for Handicapped Act
10. Externalizing
11. Executive
12. Conduct disorder
13. Panic and phobia
14. Basal ganglia
15. Boys

Multiple choice

1. d 2. a 3. c 4. b 5. c 6. b 7. a 8. a 9. a

27 ▪ *Biopsychosocial care of the elderly mentally ill*

Matching

1. g 2. h 3. i 4. j 5. a 6. f 7. b 8. e 9. c 10. d

Multiple choice

1. a 2. d 3. c 4. b 5. c 6. d 7. b 8. c

28 ▪ *Care of the homeless mentally ill*

Word unscramble

1. Deinstitutionalization
2. Chronic disaffiliation
3. Gentrification
4. Dual diagnosis
5. Homelessness

Short answer

1. Deinstitutionalization allowed many psychiatric patients to be discharged into the community, which was ill prepared to provide services for them. Many of those discharged could not meet the demands of community living without the support and supervision they had come to depend on in the hospital. Thus they became homeless.
2. Lack of affordable housing, poverty, alcohol and drug abuse, family turmoil, domestic violence, and physical or mental disability
3. Conditions exacerbated by exposure to the elements, communicable and infectious diseases that breed in crowded unsanitary conditions, trauma related to injuries associated with living on the streets, and sequelae of substance abuse
4. Asthma, pneumonia, bronchitis, and frequent colds
5. Affordable housing
6. Stigma attached to their condition, lack of insurance and transportation, lack of proof of identity, limited knowledge of available services, and fear and suspicion of service providers' agenda and fragmentation of services

Multiple choice

1. c 2. b 3. d 4. a 5. c 6. d 7. b

29 ▪ *Special care concerns for patients with dual diagnosis*

Short answer

1. Psychiatric symptoms reemerge and lead to ineffective coping, increased anxiety, substance abuse to avoid painful feelings, adverse consequences, and attempted abstinence until psychiatric symptoms emerge once more
2. Became magnified because of deinstitutionalization resulting in large numbers of homeless mentally ill living on the streets, accompanied by an increased use of drugs and alcohol
3. Primary mental illness and subsequent substance abuse, primary substance abuse disorder with psychopathologic sequelae, dual primary diagnoses, a common etiology
4. As an attempt by a person to return to homeostasis after experiencing psychological suffering, thus using alcohol or drugs to alleviate or control disturbing feelings
5. In emergency departments
6. Often, they are unreliable historians or distort reality of their mental health problems and the severity of their substance abuse
7. Their high potential for abuse
8. Substance abuse
9. Developing a relationship with persons who tend to have difficulties in their relationships and in trusting authority figures, and patients' lack of motivation and the need to encourage them to enter drug and alcohol treatment programs
10. Self-regulation, integration, understanding, self-knowledge, coping skills, change awareness, support and maintenance

Multiple choice

1. c 2. d 3. c 4. a 5. b 6. d 7. b

30 ▪ *Psychosocial aspects of medically compromised persons*

Word find

N	I	N	O	T	O	R	E	S	P	A	C	E
K	N	O	C	I	C	E	P	T	I	O	N	N
H	I	N	O	C	O	C	E	M	P	T	I	D
Y	T	N	M	S	E	R	E	P	Y	I	H	O
P	H	E	O	S	K	H	I	A	F	N	P	M
E	C	V	R	D	C	I	X	I	S	A	R	O
R	S	U	B	S	T	A	N	C	E	P	O	R
A	O	I	I	G	O	L	S	D	T	I	D	B
L	M	H	D	C	A	A	I	T	L	C	N	I
G	P	X	I	D	L	T	N	N	R	I	E	D
I	L	E	T	P	L	B	E	O	G	T	N	I
A	I	N	Y	D	O	L	L	A	M	Y	I	G

Fill in the blanks

1. Neurochemical modulation
2. Substance P
3. Serotonin
4. Hypothalamic-pituitary-adrenal (HPA) axis
5. Kindling
6. Ischemic cascade
7. Dopaminergic
8. Gate control
9. Hyperalgia, allodynia, and hyperesthesia
10. Mentation and personality

Completion exercises

First step	*Second step*	*Third step*	*Fourth step*
B, E	C, D, I	F, H	A, G

Multiple choice

1. b 2. a 3. c 4. d 5. a 6. b 7. c 8. b

31 ▪ *Biopsychosocial aspects of stress and crisis*

Matching

1. f 2. h 3. i 4. g 5. b 6. d 7. a 8. j 9. c 10. e

Sentence correction

1. Being under stress is usually viewed as a negative experience whose outcomes can be positive.
2. The person-environment relationship and cognitive appraisal are two important antecedents to the stress response.
3. True
4. True
5. True
6. Stress responses vary and are different from one person to another
7. True
8. Minimizing the seriousness of a problem is an example of emotion focused coping.
9. A crisis typically lasts no longer than 4 to 6 weeks.
10. Bereavement usually begins during a crisis.
11. True
12. True

Multiple choice

1. d 2. c 3. b 4. d 5. c 6. c 7. a 8. a 9. b 10. a

32 ▪ *Biopsychosocial management of aggression and violence*

Word unscramble

1. Assertiveness
2. Anger
3. Boundaries
4. Aggression
5. Emotional circuit

Labeling

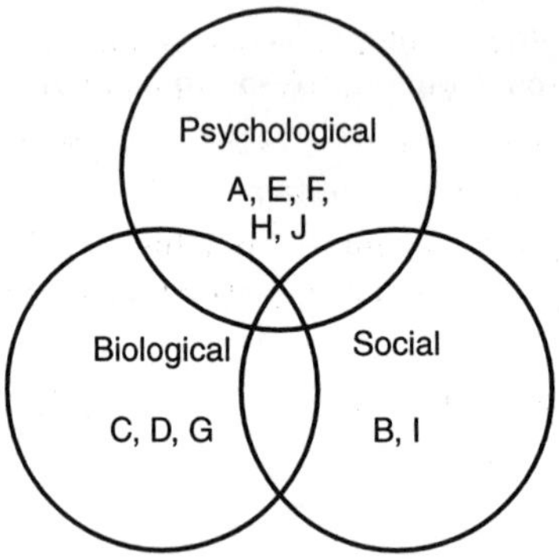

Multiple choice

1. b 2. a 3. c 4. d 5. b 6. c 7. c

33 ▪ *Biopsychosocial aspects of caring for abused persons*

Matching

1. c 2. e 3. a 4. b 5. d

Short answer

1. Devaluation of women, power inequities, and view of women as property
2. Alcohol-induced cognitive changes; drinker's expectations that alcohol increases the tendency toward aggression and sociocultural beliefs that people are not accountable for their behavior after drinking
3. Battering
4. Power imbalance and intermittency
5. The right to be a child and behave like a child; to be safe and protected from harm; and to be fed, clothed, and nurtured for growth, development, and fulfillment of child's unique potential
6. Girls often become passive, cling to others and withdraw; while boys typically become aggressive, fight with siblings and school mates and have temper tantrums
7. Older age, dependency on caregivers, alcohol abuse, history of significant intergenerational conflict between elder and caregiver, physical or mental impairment, and provocative behavior
8. Depression
9. Low self-esteem, guilt and shame, and anger
10. Traumatic bonding

Multiple choice

1. b 2. a 3. c 4. d 5. c 6. b 7. a 8. c 9. b 10. b

34 ▪ *Case finding and care in suicide: children, adolescents, and adults*

Matching

1. d 2. f 3. a 4. b 5. c 6. e

Short answer

1. a. Psychological
   b. Biologic
   c. Social
   d. Psychological
   e. Social
2. Seriousness of the person's intent, the degree to which a viable plan has been developed, availability of the measures to execute the plan
3. Aged 15 to 24 and over age 75
4. Childhood trauma, including physical and sexual abuse
5. Grief often severe and protracted; may be complicated by ambivalent feelings about the deceased; survivor may not have previous experience with suicidal death and thus lacks available coping mechanisms; extra guilt about not recognizing the impending act
6. Identify persons who may be suicidal; determine the risk for suicide; diagnose presence of psychiatric disorders, and provide for patient safety
7. Recurrent major depressive disorder, especially when comorbid with panic and severe anxiety disorders, schizophrenia, substance abuse, and borderline and antisocial personality disorders
8. Clear decision making (intent), clear and realistic method (plan), some knowledge about how to carry out the act, and no real perceived barriers to complete the act.

Multiple choice

1. b 2. a 3. b 4. d 5. c 6. a 7. b 8. a

35 ▪ *Medical emergencies in psychiatric care*

Word find

T	M	W	H	S	U	L	F	E	N	I	P	O	R	T	A	U	R	I	C
R	U	A	S	P	E	C	I	F	I	C	G	R	A	I	M	A	H	V	I
I	I	T	E	S	O	D	R	E	V	O	G	U	R	D	Y	Y	Y	I	G
C	H	E	B	A	L	T	I	Y	S	S	R	U	T	H	O	N	P	T	R
Y	T	R	S	E	R	O	T	O	N	I	N	S	Y	N	D	R	O	M	E
A	I	I	U	D	O	U	V	G	I	I	V	S	P	M	G	L	S	Y	N
I	L	A	N	R	U	I	D	E	B	Y	T	I	C	I	X	O	T	F	I
S	D	N	O	T	S	W	A	O	S	A	O	I	O	E	L	C	H	L	L
P	Y	X	L	H	T	I	L	C	Y	T	A	P	A	R	O	T	E	U	O
I	H	I	C	A	R	G	C	I	N	Z	Y	N	A	T	B	H	N	I	H
D	P	C	O	U	O	X	I	X	D	H	O	P	Y	H	I	I	U	S	C
Y	T	A	Y	Y	B	I	N	O	R	A	T	R	O	P	N	E	R	H	I
L	I	L	M	S	E	R	O	T	O	S	C	I	L	C	Y	C	I	R	T
O	O	N	O	I	T	A	C	I	X	O	T	N	I	R	E	T	A	W	N
P	S	P	E	C	I	F	I	C	G	R	A	V	I	T	Y	Z	I	M	A

Multiple choice

1. c 2. c 3. a 4. b 5. d 6. b 7. d 8. b 9. d 10. a